Chapter I

TO WHAT QUESTIONS
DOES PHENOMENOLOGY TRY TO
FIND AN ANSWER?

A PATIENT APPEARS AT THE CONSULTING HOUR OF THE PSYCHIATRIST

A FEW YEARS ago I was rung up at an unusually late hour in the evening by a man who in an obviously nervous voice asked to be allowed to consult me about his private difficulties. On my suggesting that he should come the following day in the course of the afternoon, he replied that for very special reasons he must prefer an hour in the evening. We arranged that he should come in. the evening of the day mentioned and it was indeed at the hour agreed upon that I shook hands with a young man of about 25, who told me he was the man who had rung me up and after a moment's hesitation he explained to me the reason of his visit.

Those very first moments already showed me that he was in very serious difficulties. He regarded me with a mixture of suspicion, diffidence and uneasiness and when he took my proffered hand I felt a limp hand, which did not press mine, as is frequently the case with people who do not see a way out and helplessly suffer themselves to be pushed around by circumstances. Stooping and a little uncertainly he reached the chair I had offered him.

He did not settle comfortably in his chair but left some space between himself and the back of the chair, as if he wanted to be prepared from the beginning to get to his feet and leave me. His right hand, which on coming into the room he had kept under his unbuttoned waistcoat, removing it for a moment to greet me so irresolutely, immediately slipped back into its former position. With his left hand he drummed restlessly on the arm of his chair. He left his legs uncrossed. All this gave me the impression of a man already tormented for a long time, flying before a disaster whose nature he himself does not know.

His story amply confirmed this first impression. He was an undergraduate, but had not attended any lectures for months, because he could not bear walking in the streets in broad daylight. The few times that he had forced himself to do so had remained fixed in his memory as a nightmare. He had had an ever increasing feeling that the houses he passed were about to fall down on top of him. The houses seemed to him to be drab and older than he had imagined them. They gave the impression of being dilapidated. The street had been alarmingly wide and empty and the people he had seen remained at an unreal distance. Even when a person brushed past him he had a feeling as if a great distance separated them. He felt himself grow unspeakably lonely and at the same time more and more scared. Fear forced him to return to his room and he would certainly have run if he had not been attacked by such violent palpitations of the heart that he had only been able to accomplish his return pace by pace.

He had already been troubled by attacks of palpitation for along time. At first—some years before—they were of a temporary nature and bearable, but in the long run they occurred oftener and were more violent, until at last even while there were no attacks the heart continued to beat more rapidly than he deemed natural. He constantly "felt" his heart and had to keep his hand on the cardiac region in order to ascertain continually that no irregularities occurred and also to support as it were the heart and to curb it.

He was least troubled by these disturbances in his own room. He felt best when, *undisturbed* by anybody's presence, he occupied himself with his studies. Apart from juridical and philological literature relating to his studies, he could not read any book. He had not had a novel in his hands for years and he was sure that his heart would begin to show irregularities if he did. For the same reason he could never read a newspaper. He would only allow a few friends to come to his rooms. Those were friends who spoke of nothing but science or if they touched on the usual topics of the day at all, they spoke scoffingly. Scathing talk about the female sex even restored him to a certain degree of good health. He could laugh heartily then and scarcely felt his heart. His opinion on love was correspondingly cynical. Heartily approving, he cited the definition of the French moralist, Chamfort, according to whom love was nothing but "the contact of two epiderms and the exchange of two pale fantasies."

During the time when he did not yet feel so very ill he had once been in touch with a girl. When she pressed for an engagement he had laughed her to scorn. She had sadly gone away then and he had noticed in surprise that his heart began to beat violently. He had then formed a resolution never to enter upon anything like a serious relationship with any girl again. Since that time he regularly, though not frequently, visited prostitutes, whom he humiliated in every possible way, and never touched.

About once every three months he visited his parent who lived at some 25 miles' distance. Of course he took an evening train and as a rule felt intensely miserable during the journey. On arrival he mostly became aware of a grateful feeling of rest "in his body," which disappeared again however after a couple of hours because he became increasingly annoyed at the behavior of his parents. He thought his father ill-mannered and boorish; when his mother sat down beside him and tenderly inquired after his studies, hatred flared up within him and more than once he had had to keep himself from striking her in the face. In that house, where every corner and every article of furniture recalled his youth, long past happenings came back to him and at such moments he would have delighted in hurling reproaches at his parents' heads, couched in the most scurrilous terms. He was always happy when such a weekend had come to an end. On the return journey he would find an empty compartment, where in a biting voice he cursed his life and his parents, and once back in his own room, he silenced every memory of the past by burying himself in his books.

He never thought of the future or rather he did not want to. Life did not mean much more to him than studying without any fixed purpose. If he was compelled now and then to look forward there seemed to be nothing but vagueness and fear.

2. SUMMARY OF THE PATIENT'S COMPLAINTS

We shall now pass on to a summary of the complaints that the patient expressed during his first visit, supplemented with what he added afterwards. For the purpose of surveying the complaints will be rubricated under a number of headings. Keeping as closely as possible to the patient's own story, we must state that his complaints refer to changes of the visible world, of his body, of the way in which this is related to his fellow men, of his past and of his future. If we do not wish to give a theoretical interpretation of these changes, it is better that we should, for the present, keep entirely to this classification.

a. The world

Of this world we can say that it has changed in such a way that he does not venture any more to leave the house in broad daylight. On our asking the patient what these changes are, he says that the street appeared very wide to him and that the houses gave the impression of being colorless, drab and so old and tumbledown, that he could not but expect to see them collapse at any moment. The houses also seemed to him to be very much shut up, there seemed to be shutters before all the windows, although he could very well perceive that this was not the case. He would rather have spoken of closed fortresses. When he looked up he noticed that the houses leant over towards the street, so that the strip of sky between the roofs was considerably narrower than the street in which he walked. In a square he was struck by a spaciousness that far surpassed the size of the square. He was quite certain that he would not be able to cross a square; any attempt, he suspected, would founder on such an overwhelming sense of emptiness, vast-ness, hollowness and desolation, that his legs would give way and that he would fall down. From the safe enclosure of his study the street presented a far less dangerous aspect. But also there a moment's imagining that he was standing or walking in the street was sufficient for the just mentioned feeling to force itself upon him. He had not been outside the town, in the fields or woods for years. Yet he knew very well what he would find there. His parents lived in the country, from their house he could see the fields and his bedroom even looked out on a very wide and really magnificent view. Of this splendor, which he remembered so well from former days, he had not seen anything for a long time. The colours of the flowering fields and trees did not appeal to him any more, everything looked curiously dull and lifeless. Moreover he was sure that he would be incapable of even the shortest walk.

The patient drew such a vivid picture of all this that one could not help wondering whether he was not actually living in another world, not a world designed by fiction or by a poetical imagination, but a world as real as our own, but utterly dissimilar. This impression: that the patient drew a picture of what was an absolute utter *reality* to him, grew even stronger when one saw how heavily all this weighed on him. There was no question here of a playful fancy, but of a reality, definitely guiding the patient in all his doings. It was simply impossible for him to shake off his nightmare impressions in the street: he *saw* things in that way, the things of his world were frightening and ominous and when he managed to bring himself to saying that the houses, the square, the street surely must have retained their former character and appearance and that therefore his observation must be at fault regarding what existed "in reality," then his correction would seem to him to be much more artificial than the direct, non-corrected observation that frightened him and drove him back into his rooms. What he saw was as he described it.

Let us pretend to accompany our patient on one of his walks. The day is bright, the sun is shining, people are going cheerfully along the street, which shows a friendly aspect. When we have only just left the house the patient catches hold of us, his face assumes a rigid expression, he looks anxiously about him. When we ask him what troubles him he says that the street frightens him, the houses are leaning over towards the street, he expects them to fall down. We speak to him quietly and say that on the contrary the street makes a very jolly impression, but he shakes his head and is in no way convinced. Indeed, as we walk along, he is growing more and more anxious, notwithstanding our reassuring words, so firmly founded upon "truth"; he tightly grips our arm, as if we were not giving him sufficient support, sweat stands on his forehead and it looks as if something terrible is about to happen to him. The attempt is abandoned and a few minutes later we are back again in his room. After he has recovered a little, we cannot help saying in some surprise: "Why? Surely, there was *nothing* wrong!" It is no use; the patient is not convinced by these words. On the contrary, he says that we have no notion of what he went through in the street.

It seems important to me to retain from the above the following: What to the patient is irrefutable reality, proves "on closer inspection" in our eyes not to exist at all.

b. The body

The physical complaints of the patient, who does not show any signs of physical suffering, chiefly relate to the heart. For years he has been troubled by palpitations. At first the attacks were bearable, but in course of time they became so violent that he expects to fall to the ground because of weakness. He also feels pains in the cardiac region, which persist apart from the attacks. Feeling his pulse, we are indeed struck by a too rapid and somewhat irregular rhythm. "When we tell the patient that he had better have himself examined by a heart specialist, he replies that he has already visited a number of cardiologists, all of whom assured him that not a single deviation in connection with his heart was to be found. The last cardiologist, who had advised him to consult a psychiatrist, gave him a letter. This letter proves that an exhaustive examination has been performed by a wellknown specialist, who could not discover any deviation apart from the somewhat rapid and irregular pulse. "We take from the letter an electrocardio-graphic film showing once more that there is nothing the matter with the heart. The patient knows, but is in no way convinced. He is positive that deviations would certainly be found if the methods of examination were more accurate. Cannot he personally prove the Tightness of his arguments? He has only got to walk a few steps down the street to feel in his chest how ill he is, he is convinced his heart would collapse if he were to walk any further. Besides: does not he feel his heart hurting all day? Letters from all the cardiologists in the world would fail to convince him of the non-existence of this pain or that he is not suffering from heart attacks. His heart is ill: that is the reality of his life.

He moreover complains of muscular weakness in his legs and of equilibrium disturbances. Nearly every evening after dark he goes for a short walk. In the beginning of his illness there was no trouble, however in course of time he could not manage without the support of a stout stick. Afterwards even a stick was insufficient and he discovered that he could only walk well if he had his bicycle beside him and held on to the handle-bars with both hands. Since then he has not gone out without his bicycle. Still, the people in the neighborhood are mistaken, who think that he goes for a bicycle ride every evening. He would never be able to sit on a bicycle. The mere thought causes attacks of dizziness. If the streets are slippery in winter, he stays at home. He is very careful when buying footwear: there should not be the slightest chance of losing his balance through slipping. We need hardly say that he consulted an otologist. The latter examined the patient and told him his organ of balance was unimpaired, "so" he need not worry. Alas, the trouble remained and the patient went to see a neurologist, who, however, after another exhaustive examination, declared that in his province not a single disturbance was to be found.

Here again we arrive at the conclusion; the disturbances that cause the patient so much trouble that he cannot possibly doubt their reality turn out not to exist on closer inspection, that is to say: after an objective and conscientious investigation. The patient must be mistaken. He must be deluding himself, without realizing it. For who can doubt the results of the objective scientific examination?

c. Fellow man

When the patient is questioned as to his opinion regarding people, he has a ready reply. He has no real contact with them. They irritate him. When his friends talk about everyday subjects, he considers them too naive, too optimistic or too romantic. Moreover he objects to the name of "friend." For friendship is in his opinion nothing but camouflaged egoism. Those who discuss science with him are of use to his studies, and it is only for this reason that he puts up with them. Those who speak scornfully of what are called the values of life provide him with a momentary joy. With regard to girls he is at a loss. He would like best of all to leave them entirely alone. In his opinion they are inferior beings who by preference occupy themselves with what frightens him. He regards his visits to the prostitutes as the only right kind of contact one can have with women. Love is nonsense, although he is obliged to admit— almost regretfully—that this nonsense does not leave him quite unmoved. This is proved to him by the novel, which for this reason he has ceased to read. Everything reminding him of the usual way in which people are in touch with each other must be avoided by him if he is to retain his feeble sense of rest. For this reason he never reads any newspaper either.

The people in the streets remain at a curious distance, which gives him a feeling of great desolation. Even when they brush against him on the pavement the distance remains. They move like lifeless puppets rather meaninglessly through the streets, which are wide and menaced from both sides. They make him feel uneasy, lonely, frightened and angry, all at the same time. He would love to destroy these hostile figures. Properly speaking all human beings are his enemies.

"Common sense" tells us that the patient must be mistaken also on this point. He is the victim of a tremendous misunderstanding, of which he himself is the author. For though it may also be our opinion that society is ruled for the greater part by ambition and conflicting interests, we experience just as unquestionably the proofs of true sympathy, of ready friendship and self-sacrificing love. The patient however denies this most emphatically. He enumerates without the slightest hesitation a long list of events that made it clear to. him that all love and friendship is but illusion. Our words have not the least effect on him. What appears indisputable to us, indeed "objectively" perceptible, simply proves not to exist for him at all. And what we must call a grave error, an error which must be recognizable as such to all, is to him so dearly the embodiment of truth, that *his* life is characterized by it. He lives, also as far as his relations with people are concerned, in another reality. How dearly he illustrates this reality when he tells us about the people in the street. He sees them as "hostile, meaningless puppets," separated from him by a great distance. The people are characterized by *distance*. With all the honest persuasive powers at our disposal we may argue that when people brush past one it is impossible to have a feeling of distance, it is no use: this distance is for him the way in which the presence of people makes itself felt. What in our eyes does not exist is to him unshakable reality.

d. Past and future

It is very striking how very strongly the patient resents speaking of his past. He says that he remembers only very little of his early life. But what he remembers fully justifies him to state that he was very badly brought up. His father always kept him down and very often whipped him. His mother spoiled him, she did not properly prepare him for the harshness of life. As a rule he does not think of these things. But whenever he is at home with his parents these incidents of his youth recur to his mind. In every room of his parental home he savours his youth. In his opinion his parents still treat him as a child and still repeat their former mistakes. His monthly allowance—he always has to ask for it—is insufficient. Every question his father asks him about the progress of his studies is a motion of no confidence. His father sometimes inquires after his physical condition, always in the same tone of malicious pleasure. This makes him wild and he would like nothing better than to rush off at once and never return, if it were not for his absolute financial dependence. No doubt his mother means well, but all the same he must turn away from her tender approaches. If he responded to her questionings he would very soon begin to feel small and be quite probably reduced to tears and to weep at his wretched life. But that is the very thing he has to prevent. Only when he remains cold and businesslike is life bearable for him. That is why he answers his mother with frigid, businesslike words. If she approaches him too closely he gets up and leaves the room.

Now it happened that later on I was informed from two sources about the domestic circumstances of which the patient had spoken in such black terms. One of my colleagues was on intimate terms with the parents and a friend had frequently visited the family in the days when our patient was a child. Their reports certainly gave a different impression. The father was a rather self-contained man, he was absorbed in his work, but never actually forgot his family. He was a strict disciplinarian, but certainly not hard or loveless. He had left his children quite free as to their choice of a profession and had never refused them the means with which to attain their ends. Both informants described the mother as a gentle, slightly sentimental woman, who had no doubt made her children's paths a little too smooth, though certainly not to the degree the patient had indicated. They agreed in their opinion that the parents had not committed more than the usual number of educational mistakes. Outsiders were always favourably impressed by the family. The other children were on excellent terms with their parents. As a child the patient had not been conspicuous in any way. He had not been more difficult than the others. Only during the period of adolescence had he begun to show that he was not feeling happy at home. The parents had at first regarded this as an ordinary puberal difficulty and gave him great freedom, knowing as they did that any form of discipline would work out in the wrong way. But their child had not reacted normally. They had been glad that he wanted to go to the university and hoped that the free life of an undergraduate would offer a solution for the difficulties whose true nature they did not realize. But they anxiously noticed that things were going worse and worse with him.

Here we meet again with a similar discrepancy between the judgment of the patient and that of the "objective" spectators. We are inclined to agree with the latter: does not the very satisfactory development of the other children in the same family point in an unmistakable way to the fact that the patient must be wrong? And yet, of how little avail it would be if we •were to suggest this to the patient himself! He would not be convinced at all and only be deeply disappointed at so much lack of understanding on our part. Any psychiatrist knows that he may not thus speak with his patients, if his therapy is to be successful. The same holds good for the other discrepancies ascertained before; it would be quite wrong, psychothera-peutically speaking, to tell the patient that he is mistaken in his observation of the world, that he is wrong in his opinion about his heart and that he has a very misleading idea of the people around him. Here it is our business to ascertain that the patient, also as to what he remembers of the past, deviates from what can objectively be registered and that he takes his deviating impression to be an irrefutable reality: *the truth* of his youth.

Nor is the situation any different with regard to the future. If the patient, so we should like to argue, did not permit himself to be misled by his countless mistakes, if only, we should almost be inclined to shout at him, he would open his eyes to see what the world "really" looks like, how his body is "really" sound, how the people around him for the greater part "really" have the best intentions with regard to him and how his parents "really" bestowed a very decent education on him, then the future would hold nothing but good for him. He is young, intelligent, of good family and not without means. His appearance is attractive (if only he had not such a black and scowling look!) and his manners are good. The future opens invitingly before him. But when he himself is asked where things are leading, then all the doors of the future would seem to be locked and bolted. He does not know what awaits him and can only fear the worst. He cuts short all our optimistic expectations by uttering the simple but significant words that the future is a dreadful vision.

3. QUESTIONING

In the preceding section the complaints of the patient were summarized. Again and again it proved to be possible to ascertain a contradiction between the opinion of the patient and the "facts of reality." Though it must be admitted that not every psychiatric patient is an equally dear example of such a series of contradictions, still practically every interview with a psychically sick man or woman will be a repetition of much of what we related. Any psychiatrist knows that it is not as a rule of the slightest use to point out these contradictions to the patient. On the contrary. Far too many times already he has been obliged to hear from his friends and relations that his opinions do not hold water. Such arguments were no good to him, they only irritate him. It is because he wants to hear another answer that he goes to see the psychotherapist. And he does get another answer. Let us briefly state what is the train of thought of the psychotherapist.

When the patient tells him that he sees the houses as being old and tumbledown, that he, when he looks up in the street, sees that they lean over dangerously, that the fields are less alive and colorful, in short, that his world *looks different,* then the psychotherapist will not for one moment share the patient's belief that the things, the objects themselves, have changed. He considers his own perception to be right and the patient's wrong. The latter must be mistaken, on that point he is in per- feet accord with the friends and relations. But he does not say that the patient is mistaken. Not only because he knows that by telling him so the patient will be irritated. In a sense the patient is right. There has indeed been a change. But this change bears no reference to the outside world. It is the patient himself, his subject, that is psychically ill, that is to say "different." The patient is mistaken as to the locality of the change. The psychotherapist is convinced that the patient transfers his disturbed state of mind to the things he sees. In professional words: the patient *projects.* What after all really only exists *within him,* is conveyed by him to the things of his daily existence: *pro-jection.*

We have gradually become familiar with the idea of "projection." So familiar, that we no longer see the theoretical difficulties contained in this idea. Still nobody has been able to make it clear yet how a projection takes place. It is right to remember that there does not exist any single moderately feasible theory that would make it clear to us that an abnormal state of mind, a psychical disturbance, i.e., something that is present *in* the patient and nowhere else, <u>can</u> move out of him and so closely attach itself to things, can so become merged into things, that the patient sees the change as an unquestionable reality. We may be sure of one tiling: the world of which the patient speaks is as real to <u>him</u> as our world is real to us. We might almost say that to him it is even more real than to us: whereas we can successfully shake off the influence that an oppressive landscape has on us, the patient cannot. In the case we described thf patient even stayed at home in order to be no longer frightened by the things that he would see in the street.

Whoever tries to form a clear notion of what is meant by the idea of "projection" must admit that he is faced with a mystery.

Follow the physical complaints. Of course the psychotherapist agrees with the friends and relations that the body of the patient is in good health. Letters and reports from various specialists will have swept away the last remnants of doubt that he might still harbour. But he does not arrive at the too easy conclusion that the patient is suffering from an imaginary illness. The patient is ill, that is a fact. But he is ill in a way different from what the patient assumes himself: not physically but psychically. He conveys his psychical illness to the organs of his body. This conveying, this turning from psychical into physical he calls *conversion*. The patient converts.

We have here the second idea which has gradually become so well known in psychiatry that one is apt to use it unthinkingly. Do we actually realize that this idea is almost as obscure as the idea of "projection"? Let us look a little more closely to see what is meant by this term. As a rule the reasoning is as follows. Man has a body and a soul. These are essentially different. In contradistinction to the soul the body is visible and dissectible, it is a thing. The soul, such is the general, opinion, must exist somewhere within this thing. On attempting to discover this soul within this body, uncommonly little is found however. We know, it is true, that certain organs are necessary to preserve the psyche. The heart is such an organ, the brain another; and it is the latter which is very particularly allied with the existence of what we mean by the word "soul." But when we begin to dissect these organs, we don't encounter thoughts anywhere, nor desires or memories, nor fear, hope, hatred or love. It will be said that this need not surprise us: has not a definition been given beforehand that the soul is invisible and indissectible, i.e., that it has no space? But in this case it is not correct to assume that the soul should be *in* the body. What has no space cannot be *inside* or *outside* anything. The view that man has a body and a soul is in the end not comprehensible to anybody. It follows that also the difference between psychical and physical will be obscure. And he who says that psychical disturbances manifest themselves through the body really ignores a problem that cannot even approximately be solved.

But all the same let us suppose that such a thing as "the psyche" is housed somewhere in the body, how in the world are we to imagine a way in which this immaterial psyche influences the matter of the body? One remembers how thinkers such as Descartes and Leibnitz already cudgelled their minds in vain about this point. It is not indeed even in the slightest way imaginable that a "soul," considered to be non-physical, should influence the organs of the material body. Leibnitz already arrived at this conclusion, and on the strength of it propounded the astonishing theory that the soul and the body, beginning at their creation, go their own ways as two completely separate self-contained systems, ways rendered so faultlessly parallel by the Creator, that we, deceived by appearances, continually assume that they are in touch. There will not be anyone left now who still believes in this theory. No more than there is anybody to be found who thinks with Descartes that the pineal gland should have to be taken as the inconceivable metaphysical, one might almost say occult bridge, between the physical and the non-physical. Just as few people have any confidence in the artifice of the materialists and psychical monists, who get rid of the difficulty by quite simply denying either the soul or the body.

It will be said: is it for a psychiatrist to puzzle about these philosophical problems? There is something wrong though with this question. The psychiatrist speaking of conversion ought to know that in using this term he regards as solved a number of problems that are really surrounded by great obscurity. It is right that he should realize that he could never have spoken of conversion, if it had not been brought home to him that man has a body and a soul, that the soul lives in the body and is constantly in touch with this body. As soon as philosophy arrives at a more acceptable definition of man, this will mean the end of the idea of conversion. In its place there will then come as well a more acceptable interpretation of the fact that psychiatrically disturbed persons can have physical complaints. Phenomenology believes that it is able to give this better interpretation. It is true, it starts from a different philosophical definition of man, from a different anthropology. In the next chapter we shall try to describe this new anthropology in a few brief words.

But let us return for a moment to the view so generally accepted at present that the patient converts. If this were really the case, that the disturbances were not physical but wholly psychical in character, how is it then that the patient puts the full stress on his being physically out of order? We mean this: it would be more acceptable if the patient mentioned his purely psychical difficulties first and after that "their effect" on his body. What we see however is quite the reverse. Certainly, the patient "feels ill." but this "feeling" is always meant in a physical sense. He has palpitations, a heavy feeling in his epigastrium, a band round his forehead, a heaviness pressing on his head, weakness in his legs, fatigue in his arms, dizziness in his head, etc. Occasionally we get the impression that he speaks of "purely psychical complaints"; he is nervous, frightened and irritated. But he measures his nervousness by the "agitated feeling in his chest," by the "pressure on his throat" and by the "tremblings of his fingers, his hands, his whole body"; he singularly often localizes his fear in the cardiac region, his general dissatisfaction with life is identified with a bad taste in his mouth and with a sensation of nausea in his throat. Are not we led here to suspect that there is something wrong with the idea of *conversion?*

Let us now consider along what lines the psychotherapist thinks when the patient tells him that he is on bad terms with the others. We may first state that he is not any more inclined than the relations of the patient are, to believe the patient's statements. It cannot be true that nearly everybody means to harm him. He has a wrong impression of people. He is mistaken when he thinks that everybody has sinister designs upon him, that all men infringe on his personal liberty and that all girls are despicable creatures, painfully and needlessly upsetting him by their physical attractions. But how has the patient arrived at this very unfortunate misapprehension? Not infrequently does the psychotherapist give a decisive answer to this question. He says that the patient's difficulties in reality only concern his parents. During his youth something went wrong, his education did not really tend to help him to mature, but on the contrary put a brake on his development. Relations between his father and himself have become strained, he is in continual conflict with this father, but for some reason he has shifted the battHng-ground of this struggle to his contact with other men. As regards his mother, in his youth he had to wage battles against his mother's indulging, therefore too-binding love. He did not carry off the victory. He did not free himself of his mother's dominating power over him, nor of that of his father. He also ceased to struggle with his mother. But what remained thus unfinished he could not leave behind. He must fight on and he does fight on. But instead of freeing himself of his mother in this struggle, he fights duels with all the women he encounters. He *transfers* those feelings which after all only concern his parents to the rest of the world. He is the victim of *transference.*

Here we encounter a third conception, which in present-day psychiatry has become almost a commonplace: *transference,* i.e., the carrying over *(trans-ferre)* of feelings and contact difficulties bound up with these feelings from *one* person to *another,* the former being the one with whom the patient's difficulties *really* used to be concerned, while the latter is not concerned with these difficulties at all in one way or another. It is above all the psychotherapist who sees the most striking examples. For is not he himself very often the man to whom the patient transfers his feelings? Early or late, it is he for whom the patient will entertain the feelings that in last analysis are concerned with other people. The psychotherapist is hated, though he never added fuel to this hatred. He is violently loved, though on the face of it there is so little reason for such love. In the course of the treatment the reason for the behaviour of the patient is usually explained. His hatred for instance bears a close resemblance to that which he entertained towards his father, his mother, his elder or younger brother or sister. His love is a copy of that which he felt for one of the persons belonging to his youth, which led however to disappointment or to hopeless failure. What came to grief in former days is taken up again and continued in the room of the psychotherapist. This does not disturb the psychotherapist in the least. Is not he on the contrary in this way oSered the very means to relieve the patient of his morbid condition? He affords the opportunity for the patient to discharge his pent up feelings and to get rid of the misunderstanding in which he is so obviously involved. The affective history of the patient, which it was impossible to complete in daily life, finds its proper conclusion in the room, of the psychotherapist. The treatment of the patient proves to consist in the treatment of the transference. No indeed, it is impossible for the psychotherapist to doubt the existence of the *transference.* The patient recovers: this seems to him to be the proof of the soundness of his views.

In spite of this conclusive evidence for the *practical* correctness of the idea of transference, we may ask ourselves here what the situation is in connection with the more theoretical reflections forming the foundation for this conception. For it is quite possible that the interpretation of a conception giving excellent practical results consists in a theoretical error.

The best thing is to start from a simple example. In his youth a patient has learned to hate his mother, because she did not leave him free in any way. Today he hates all women. The usual line of thought is the following: the patient switches his hatred from his mother over to the others. This supposes that a feeling, in this case hatred, can be detached from the object hated. There would be then such a thing as "hatred as such." If we wish to adhere to this experience however, we shall on closer inspection be obliged to conclude that this "hatred as such," this objectless hatred was never experienced or observed. Nobody can boast of having hated without his hatred having an objective. Neither do we know of "direction-less love." In saying so we repeat Brentano's statement, which has rightly become famous, in his *Psychology* of 1874, that there exists no feeling without there being at the same time an object to which this feeling is directed. This true observation however upsets the seemingly so simple interpretation of the transference. There *must* exist such a thing as transference: there are too many and too convincing practical proofs, but that which the name suggests cannot be true. Whoever doubts this would do well to put himself in the place of him who practises transference. He who hates his mother feels this hatred to be permeated with his mother. It is impossible for him to separate his hatred from the mother to whom this hatred is directed. These two are one.

It is not hard to find an answer to the question as to how we arrived at this faulty reasoning. The cause is that we are accustomed to treat psychical qualities as if they were *things*. He who says that a feeling can be transferred from one person to another, speaks as if it were a question of carrying an ashtray from the table to his writing-table. This is all very well for things. But feelings are not things. We cannot therefore take them away from one place and put them down in another. The idea of transference is still part and parcel of physics. If it is to mean something in psychology—extensive practising of psychology favours this idea—then it will have to be defined psychologically first. But no serious attempt to find such a definition was made in psychopathology until recently.

We said before that every psychotherapist discovers with nearly every treatment that the origin of the patient's feelings is to be found in his youth. Let us turn our attention for a moment to the way in which patients see their youth and to the theoretical difficulties that present themselves.

The first thing that strikes us is that almost all neurotic patients when speaking of their youth grre a poor account of it. In nearly every case the educators seem to have been people with but little aptitude for their task. The patients report sad things: the father beat them cruelly and often, the mother was either heartless or she loved them foolishly. Occasionally an absolutely criminal occurrence is brought under consideration: the father threatens to cut off his little son's penis, if he should persist in playing with it. In the early days of modern psycho-therapeutic history these and similar reports were readily believed by the psychotherapists. They spoke of psychotraumata and would from these account for the entire neurosis. Afterwards when it became dear that there was some need for scepticism, the original doctrine of psychotraumata was abandoned. We know that already Freud and after him C. G. Jung even much more pronouncedly, both of them convinced of the erroneousness of the report given by the patients of their youth, moved back the psychotraumata to the pristine ages of mankind. It is difficult to dispute this hypothesis, because of a complete absence of any control. If there was at first a notion that there was a possibility of such a control by means of studying the customs and habits of primitive peoples, a closer acquaintanceship with these peoples has made us very careful. It is curious that it is the ethnologists who are the sharpest critics with regard to the depth-psychological hypothesis. Anyhow, we are faced with the difficult)- that the patient gives an account of his life which in no way tallies with the real facts.

Here again the psychotherapist takes the side of the friends and relatives: the patient must be mistaken. If he were not, it would be incomprehensible that in the same family other children grew up without there being any question of a neurosis. And as regards our patient: a reliable heteroanamnesis from two sides prevents us from believing that the parents really acted as the patient would have us believe. Neither however does the psychotherapist merely state here that the patient is mistaken. Following the French psychiatrist Dupre he will say that the patient is the victim of a *mythification* of his past, brought about by his neurosis. Does he realize however that his words are in contradiction with the general conception of memory, shared very probably by himself? Remembering, it is generally-said, is the recalling into consciousness of *engrammata* fixed in the brain. When I experience something, when I observe something for instance, then a memory picture of what was observed is stored away in the brain. This process is usually regarded as being purely physiological. During the observation the lens of the eye constructs a true picture of what was observed; this picture is, equally truly, guided via certain channels to those centres of the central nervous system where k can be anchored. To remember is to go back to this anchorage. This may of course be accompanied by disturbances. For instance it may happen that memory fails to properly mark off the original anchorage, memory is then contaminated with "associations" with other memories, etc. In most cases of this description we have a more or less distinct suspicion that disturbances are taking place. We then say that we can only vaguely remember, that we "cannot recall the thought" or that memory fails us. In these cases we expect that we can succeed in correcting this disturbance when "things are clear in our mind again" or when someone who was with us at the time of observation or experience "helps us to remember."

Nothing of the kind is observed in the patient. If we take the trouble, armed perhaps with reports of "eye witnesses" to cure him of his "errors," then not infrequently he would seem to cling with redoubled conviction to what we call his erroneous memory. How are we to form an idea of the possibility of such a thing, if we are to stick to the theory of the engrammata? What is the use of speaking of a mythifkation here? Can engrammata be overlaid with a myth? And, supposing that the latter could be made plausible in a way, bow then is *it possible* that the patient takes the myth to be reality and has not the faintest suspicion of the tremendous mistake he makes? If it were only possible to assume that the patient intentionally deceives us. But we soon abandon this idea when we speak with him. No, we may be sure of one thing: the patient is in perfectly good faith.

The patient is in good faith. On our asserting this, some psychotherapists will interrupt us and say that the deception practised by the patient exists without the shadow of a doubt, but remains *unconscious*. And the opponents will go on to say that the same holds good for all the contradictions noted above. The patient lives in a world that differs from ours, he projects his subjective condition into the happenings of his daily life, but this *projection takes place unconsciously*. The patient has physical disturbances that cannot be verified by any medical examination, he converts, *but converts unconsciously*. The patient is quite convinced of the hostility or the affection of the people around him, in spite of the fact that as far as we can see those people have not shown the slightest sign. He is the victim of transference, *but this transference takes place unconsciously*.

All at once this would seem to make everything perfectly acceptable again. Indeed it is not so very hard to stick to the above criticized conceptions of projection, conversion, transference and mythiflcation, if at the same time the hypothesis of *the unconscious* is set up. The method is very simple. With every theoretical difficulty a new quality is attributed to the unconscious eliminating the difficulty. When we for instance ascertain that hatred as such, objectless hatred, is never experienced and that the unconscious is exactly that faculty of man within which objectless feelings do occur, within which therefore a feeling can be separated from its original object and which consequently allows transferring to another object, then the sting is taken out of our criticisms. The more so, because there is no possibility of control whatever. For is not the unconscious defined as exactly that which eludes our attention? The unconscious is never experienced, so in an appeal to experience there is no sense at all.

Yet one objection remains. The lines of thought accompanying the ideas of projection, conversion, transference and mythi-fication were proved just now to have a very bad case psychologically or even to be unacceptable. Can these lines of thought be preserved by a new hypothesis which definitely turns away from the province of actual psychology? For once more: the unconscious has never been experienced. As soon as it is experienced it stops being unconscious. Many psychopathologists have felt unhappy about this point They felt like a physicist who hears that unsolved physical problems have been unraveled by means of the occult sciences.

The phenomenologist sees the hypothesis of the unconscious as a too rapid, premature swerving away from the solving of the theoretical difficulties presented by the psychiatrical patients. He stands fascinated by the curious discrepancy existing between the opinions of the patient and "actual reality." Before surrendering to the theory of the unconscious he wants to enter very fully into the nature of the above mentioned discrepancies. For this purpose he puts the following questions: a. What is the relationship of man and his *ivorld* and what is to be said of this relationship when man is psychically disturbed? b. What is the relationship of man and his *body* and what is to be said of this relationship when man is psychically disturbed? c. What is the relationship of man and *fellow men* and what is to be said of this relationship when man is psychically disturbed? d. What is the relationship of man and his past or, putting it more generally, *time,* and what is to be said when man is psychically disturbed? After which he finally puts this question to himself: is there any need of setting up the hypothesis of an unconscious psychical life, of *"tb4* unconscious?*

In the following chapter an attempt will be made to set forth the answers as they are to be found in present-day phenomenologkal psychology and psychopathology.

Chapter II

THE ANSWERS

I. MAN AND WORLD

IT IS WINTER. Evening is falling and I get up to switch on the light. Looking out of the window I see that it has begun to snow. Everything is getting covered by the sparkling snow, which is falling down silently from the heavily overcast sky. People move soundlessly past my window. I hear a man stamping the snow from his boots. I rub my hands and look forward to the evening that is to follow. For a few days ago I rang up a friend to ask him to come and spend this evening with me. In about an hour's time he will arrive at my house. Now that it is snowing outside the evening becomes even more attractive to me. I bought a bottle of good wine yesterday, which I place at the proper distance from the brightly burning fire. I sit down at my desk to write some letters. Half an hour later the telephone rings. It is my friend to tell me that he is unexpectedly prevented from corning. We talk for a moment and arrange for another day. When I lay down the telephone it seems as if my room has become somewhat quieter. The hours that follow seem emptier and longer to me. I throw some logs on the fire and settle down at my desk again. A few minutes later I am engrossed in a book, lying before me. The evening slips slowly away. When I lift my head to reflect on a passage that refuses to become quite clear, my eye is caught by the bottle standing by the fire. I realize once more that my friend has not come and then return to my book.

Surveying this episode, taken from everyday life, we may perceive that there are constant reactions between the subject and his surroundings. I expect my friend, I render this *sub jective* situation visible to myself by changing the *things* in my room: I light the fire, put cigarettes ready to hand and warm the wine. To others too the subjective situation has become clear; anyone entering unexpectedly would most probably exclaim: I see you are expecting company to-night! I notice that it is snowing; this *objective* situation is evidently capable of strengthening extraordinarily my *subjective* expectation. When the telephone has removed my *expectation* it has become quieter *in my room*. When afterwards I <u>refer</u> sight of the bottle, this *objective* fact makes me realize anew that my *subjective* expectation was dashed to the ground.

We shall now be glad to know the truth about this reaction. In order to attain this aim we concentrate on the last fact (: I see the bottle of wine standing there and reali2E that my friend stayed away), and ask this question: *What do 1 see when I notice this bottle?* The answer would seem very simple. I see a green bottle with a white label, on which is printed the name of a brand. On looking closer I can read the printed words. It is a bottle of Medoc. The bottle is corked and a lead capsule has been fixed over the closure. I can go on and enumerate all the details of the bottle. What becomes rapidly clear to rne however is that in this way I shall certainly not come nearer to what happened when looking up I saw the bottle standing there. What I saw was very definitely not green glass, white label, lead capsule, etc. What I saw in reality, well, that was something like a disappointment that my friend had not come, the loneliness of my evening. Of course I saw a bottle, but my seeing instantly meant that I passed the thing bottle over to the value which this bottle had acquired for me.

The positivistic psychologist will no doubt rebuke me and say that this is too poetical an explanation. He informs me that it really was a glass bottle with a label that I saw, but that this observation was contaminated with the projection of my subjective condition: my disappointment and my loneliness. But I don't give in. If it were my projection I saw. should not I see my loneliness more dearly then, and less complicatedly, if I did not ask the question of the bottle, but asked myself what my feelings were? An *introspection* would show me even much more convincingly what my feelings are. Well, nothing of all this is the case in reality. Asking myself by means of introspection how things are with me, then, my sense of loneliness is much less vividly revealed to me.

Another example. A married couple, that visited Paris on their honeymoon, go to the same city on a holiday trip ten years later. In the train they recollect numerous incidents. Palis comes to life for them again. But what Paris meant to them in those days becomes only clear to them when they go down the stairs of the *Metro* and inhale the typical smell of the Paris subway. The introspection that took place in the train gave them a memory which may be called a dim reflection of the memory which apparently comes to meet them with the smell. Are not we invited to assume that the memory, this *subjective* condition *par excellence,* is tied up in a smell of the Metro, so in an *object?*

Von Uexkuell and Kriszal give an example in their book on the *World of Man and Animal* (1954) which is certainly to the point here. They ask how different people see one and the same oak. To the huntsman the oak is a shelter for the game and a cover for himself, to the wood merchant the oak is a measurable, countable and saleable object, the young romantic girl sees in the same oak a facet of a love landscape. They see absolutely different things. And yet, don't they see exactly the same oak all the same? Is not there a curious contradiction here? We shall always go on thinking this a curious contradiction if we don't distinguish two forms of observation. If we mean by observation an objective, scientific inspection, then indeed the three persons mentioned see exactly the same: an oak, a tree shaped in a special way with a trunk, branches, leaves and fruit. But with this kind of observation psychology has extremely little to do. Usually man observes in a very different way. He seldom sees objects, things as such, he sees *significations* which things assume for him. He, we should like to put it, understands the language that things speak to him. If he does not understand this language in any way. then he does not observe anything either. It is certain that the romantic girl notices things in the oak absolutely unsuspected by the wood merchant; he in his turn notices details non-existent for the girl. One day an inhabitant of Malacca, who had never seen anything outside his village and the jungle, was suddenly taken to Singapore and shown a large part of this metropolis. When at the end of the tour he was asked what had struck him, he never mentioned, as he had been expected to do, the paved streets, stone houses, cars, trams and trains., but he said that it had surprised him that one single man could carry so many bananas. What he had seen appeared to be in the first place a banana seller, who could transport so many bunches of bananas in his cart. For the rest he had hardly noticed anything; since cars and stone houses could not acquire any *signification* for him, he had noticed them very little or not at all.

What a man sees, hears, tastes and smells in the very first place concerns himself. The huntsman sees his intention to hunt, i.e., his subjective intention, when the oak shows itself to him as a possibility for taking cover; the wood merchant shows himself what he is, when he sees in the oak a trunk, i.e., future boards; the girl proves her romantic love, when she sees the oak in her own way. Similarly I realize so to say my disappointment, when I see the bottle of wine standing by the fire and the couple, married for ten years, recollect the Paris of their honeymoon when they smell the scent of the underground.

If we want to get to know a man, we had better not inquire into his introspective-observable "subjective" state. As a rule the answer is singularly insignificant. We only gain an insight into the nature of his subjectivity, when we make him describe the objects, when we asJc him to give us a description of his world. Not the world as "on closer inspection" it turns out to be, but the world as it is seen by means of that other, immediate., living, daily observation. The "closer inspection" destroys the reality of our existence. It was this "closer inspection" which has so greatly handicapped the development of psychology.

Of all this the present-day psychologist and psychopathologist need hardly be told. He refrains by preference from asking "how things are with a person," because he knows that the answer will be irrelevant. He resorts to putting a number of pictures before a person and asks him to speak of what he sees.

And then it is of no interest to him what the patient sees "on closer inspection": a man in trousers, waistcoat, etc., no, he gauges the original observation by asking the patient what is happening, he tries to find the *signification* which the things in the picture have for the patient. He never learns to know the *subject* better than by *going* to the *objects,* to the things of his world.

We can summarize all this *as* follows. The relationship of man and world is so profound, that it is an error to separate them. If we do, then man ceases to be man and the world to be world. The world is no conglomeration of mere objects to be described in the language of physical science. The world is our home, our habitat, the materialization of our subjectivity. Who wants to become acquainted with man, should listen to the language spoken by the things in his existence. Who wants to describe man should make an analysis of the "landscape" within which he demonstrates, explains and reveals himself.

It is my duty towards the great number of those who will probably consider the above as well as the following remarks too "philosophical" to add a few words to these statements . The rigid separation of man and world is by no means the fruit of a course of thought naturally proper to man. This separation too is the result of purely philosophical reflection. It was Descartes, who in purely philosophical writings cut a deep cleft between man and world, between non-dimensional and dimensional "things," between what he called the *rel cogitantes* and the *ret extensae*. Since then this separation has been applied in all regions of thought even to extreme limits It is easily understood that this was greatly to the benefit of the physical sciences. It should be as easy to understand that it was as greatly to the detriment of such a science as psychology. What we have seen since the days of Descartes consists indeed in an ever increasing expansion of the physical sciences, whereas psychology deviated ever more in the direction of physiology. We now live in an age which the Dutch psychologist Hermans has, not without reason, called the age of psychology. Is it so much to be wondered at that this age opened with Husserl's very severe criticism of Descartes' philosophical theory?

When Freud in his famous *Drei Abhandlungen zur Sexual-theorie* postulates that libido arises *in* the subject, independent of the stimuli of the world, then it is right to consider that this remark could not possibly have flown from his pen if Descartes had not argued before him that man is a subject completely foreign to the world. And whoever adheres with Freud and so many other psychologists to the theory of projection, has unwittingly voted for a very definite philosophical view of man and world. Four centuries of scientific tradition have resulted in our no longer noticing the philosophical foundation of our way of *seeing* and consequently also of *thinking.* In the twentieth century it appears that this way of seeing and thinking leads to contradictions, to unsolvable psychological problems. There is every reason therefore for asking what the situation is of our implicit philosophy. This questioning cannot be done otherwise than philosophically.

The first result of this philosophical reflection consists in a new definition of the relationship of man and the world. A new light is seen to fall on the signification of the complaints of the patients.

In his *Studien zur Pathogenese* (1935) V. Von Weizsacker tells of a patient, a lady, suffering from *diabetes insipidus.* Of course her complaint consists in the subjective state of continual thirst. But it would be a mistake to think that this thirst shows itself to her solely or even principally as a state subjectively perceptible. She expresses her disturbance as follows: "I feel akin to water. I swim whenever and wherever I find an opportunity. I often think that it is definitely beautiful when a powerful jet of water is made to flow in at the neck. I love brooks, that is why I always go to the Black Forest. When I am there, I look for the paths skirting a brook. Water is purity." That she is ill, is different, means in the first place to her that she sees the world differently. If we want to know how she experiences her illness, i.e., how this illness strikes her, we should receive but a scanty report, if we asked her how she feels subjectively. We only gain a good idea of *her* change, when we ask how the world looks to her.

Here arises an "extrospective pathograpby." A pathography that does not stop at enumerating what the patient introspectively can observe "in himself" as "conscious state," but which consists in a description of the pathological *physiognomy of the world* (Erwin Strauss), i.e., in the description of those changes that are also to the patient most immediately noticeable and most convincing.

When waking up after a broken night, one perceives that one is ill and decides to spend a day in bed, then of course on being asked, one can give an account of the state of illness by saying that there is a feeling of fatigue and heaviness, that one has no appetite and is suffering from a dull headache. But a real description of the subjective state of illness is not given before one tells of the wallpaper looking so different, that the telephone has a different sound, more distant, less real, how the sounds made by the cars in the street, the voices of people outside, penetrate into the room where the patient lies in an entirely new way. To be ill, says the chronic heart patient, Pastorelli, who, in her *Servitude et grandeur de la maladie* (1933), has given us an excellent description of a sickbed ending in death, to be ill means in the very first place that one's surroundings have dunged in some discouraging way, it means that also one's best friends recede to a hopeless distance, that the world of human activities calls urgently, as never before, for one's pattidpatian, now become quite impossible. To be ill means to the patient in the first place a new, sick physiognomy of the world.

It is especially the psychically disturbed patients who tell us so spontaneously. The depressed person says that the world has become grayer. The colors of the flowers have faded, the sunlight is less brilliant. One of my patients even came to buying new incandescent lamps, because the light in his room had grown so much dimmer in the evening. The maniac sings the praises of the world, which never before showed itself to him in such loveliness and colors. And the incipient schizophrenic everywhere sees, hears and smells the indications of an approaching world catastrophe, the end of the world. He smells the sulphorous fumes already rising from the earth, he can tell by people's voices and the blowing of the wind that the ominous change is due, the taste of the bread he eats speaks of a diabolic poison impregnating the things of this world. We would certainly not understand all this very clearly if we said that it is "only fancy," "projection," "nothing but a metaphor." The patient is ill, this means at once that the world is ill; while telling what his world looks like, he tells us without prevarication, without any mistake, *how he is himself*.

Let us now return to the patient of the first chapter. He says that the houses look old and tumbledown, he observes that they are on the point of collapsing, the)' lean over towards him as if they would crush him. The phenornenologist wants to take it all literally. The street where the patient goes *is* like that. The street, it is true, is not so to us, but this only means that the patient is ill and we are not. Nothing gives us the right to regard our perception as being more true than that of the patient. It is also our perception that proves to us how and what we are, If we find that our opinions much resemble those of innumerable others, it only means that the people surrounding us are for the greater part psychically in good health and that they grew up in a similar cultural world. For if we make a Pygmy or a Tibetan walk down the same street, they, notwithstanding their psychical health, see a very different street. We need not even go so far afield : the peasant, the ocean fisherman and the working man of our own country, when going down the same street, also see streets widely differing from each other. A woman, a man, a small child, an adolescent and an aged person also observe other streets. They see their age, their descent, their education, their family, their profession and their intelligence. These qualities of the subject are in the first place aspects of the world, physiognomies of the things of their daily existence.

The patient demonstrates his condition. His existence really verges on a collapse, everything pertaining to him really is old and decrepit: he lives with the relics of a time that has vanished, he is a living anachronism. That the streets and squares are terrifyingly wide and empty to him is the literal expression of his subjective state. He is a lonely unit and lacks the contacts with living reality, things are distant, foreign and hostile to him. He could not have described his condition better, he gives us a true picture of his psychical illness.

For the first time in the history of psychiatry the psychiatrist does not side with the layman., with the relatives and friends. He does not form his opinion of the patient too hastily, but he puts himself in his place, i.e., in his world. The opinion of the layman is always a condemnation. In accordance with this was the nomenclature: a vocabulary of denigrations, however good the intention. The patient was said to have black moods, he is melancholy: his feelings are a blade, minus-variant of ours; or he had run off the rails: bis behaviour lacked the efficient brakes that form part of our perfect, healthy life. They spoke of hyperesthesia, hypeAiucsc, hyperthymia, hypobulimy or of hypomnesia and bypofvocesu.. The patient suffered of a too much or a too tittie, he sinned so to say in being different, he was a dissonance. Dementia, amorality, penrusitf, imbecility and idiocy strike, if possible, an even stronger note of condemnation. His life was a mass of errors. And of mistakes: he projected, which we, the healthy, do only by way of exception and had better avoid. Does not all this form part of the times when the mental patients were condemned and locked up? I am exaggerating, for our attitude towards the patient has greatly changed since those days and changed for the better. My plea would be however that our nomenclature should not be condemnatory any longer either. It is not of any importance to ascertain that the patient is not as we are. Even the layman knows as much. But it is important to know the nature of his existence. The pathography should not bear a negative but a positive character: we wish to know the nature of the existence that the patient leads, we wish to know what his world looks like.

2. MAN AND BODY

R. L. Stevenson in his fascinating novelette *The bottle imp* tells of a man whom life has treated well. With the help of the magic spirit dwelling in the bottle he has become a rich man. He has bought a delightful house in one of the sunny islands of the Pacific and has married a good, thoughtful, loving wife. On waking up in the morning he leaves his bed singing and singing he washes his healthy body. One morning his wife suddenly hears his song stopped short. She goes to see what is the matter and discovers her husband in a state of distraction and dismay. By way of explanation he points to a small spot on his body, a pale spot: he has leprosy. The discovery of this apparently very slight change has knocked over his whole life. It interests him no longer that he is a rich man, possessing one of the finest houses in the world. He has no eyes any more for the splendour of the island. This splendour is lost on him, if anything it intensifies his despair. A few moments before his thoughts went out to his wife with love and longing, but now she belongs to the caste of the healthy, now to be out of his reach forever.

This discovery is made every year by thousands upon thousands of people. The woman who, busy at her toilet, feels "the small lump in her breast," puts down the soap and tells herself the shattering news that death has forced an entrance into her life. The man who suffered for a few months with obstipation and hears the doctor speak of the necessity of a serious operation, sees that the setting of the stage of his Life is being altered. Would not these people be highly surprised to hear that the body is nothing but an anonymous, purely material husk of what man really is, his soul? Do we ourselves, the healthy, believe in this theory so strongly dominating our medical and psychological mode of thought implicitly or even explicitly? Do not we live with the reality, the same reality which so convincingly dominates the physical sick, *thai u'e are our body?* He who perceives that a malignant disease has attacked his body, surely does not console himself with the remark that his illness is only concerned with his physical shell; he knows that his whole existence, *his psychical life* has been struck by a calamity. The worried mother who is sitting by the bedside of her sick child and caresses his little arm, does definitely not caress a sheath which is supposed to hold her child, but she touches the child itself, the caressing contact of hand and arm is the contact of two human beings, without any barrier, direct. The young woman who tends her body and prepares herself for the encounter, cleanses and tends not a thing between herself and the world, between herself and the other, an obstacle as it were, she tends *herself.* We might continue in this way. There are examples without number, furnishing so many proofs, that man is identical with his body.

This is not likely to be disputed. But there will be many who would add that man *has* a body as well. Quite correct. A simple example will suffice. I can look in the glass and ascertain that I *have* a curious face. Whoever would be inspired to do so, can even cut off a finger and throw it to us with the words; I *had* it, I now *have* it no longer. Nobody will deny that this is not exactly an everyday occurrence. Who says that he *bos* a body, has in fact removed himself already from his normal existence. Looking in the glass, we usually say: "I am plain" or "I am handsome"; this is already a great deal more usual than to say: the face I have is plain, etc. Nor will anybody conclude his examination at the glass with the words; "I must shave ofi the hair stubbles from the face I have." We say: "I must wash *myself,*" "I must cut *my* nails." He who in daily life speaks of his body would seem to be speaking about himself.

We come upon a curious thing here, which we also encountered in much the same form during the discussion of the reiatiooship of man and world. Could we ascertain at the time that thought, *reflection,* creates a distance between man and world which in daily life, hence before all thought: *"pre~reflec-tiiel."* is not to be found; here, with the discussion of the relationship of man and body, we must say just as positively that the two *" pre-reflecttvely"* are, if not identical, yet very closely related, whereas reflection discloses an enormous difference. From this reflection arises Descartes' conviction that our body belongs to the world of the dimensional things, of the *rei exten-sae,* in which we ourselves have no share at all. Descartes' opin- ion has been extraordinarily fertile for medical science. For a "thing" that we "have" we can analyze and through this try to explain. Whereas that which we *are* can properly speaking not be analyzed. The medical student who caresses the hand of his fiancee commits an unpardonable fault when he repeats his anatomy at the same time. The hand of the girl he loves *has no* blood vessels, muscles, nerves and bones. Even the physiologist knows that it is indecent and untrue to speculate at a festive board on the fate of the food he takes; he does not convey food to his mouth: he (not his body) *eats* together with others. Nor do most complicated chemical processes take place in his stomach: he perceives that in an agreeable way he is being satisfied, In "pre-reflective" life, i.e., in life as we ordinarily live it, we have not the stomach of the textbook, but rather, while eating, we ourselves have *become* stomach, just as while studying we *become, are* head, are head to such an extent that we do not notice the craving of the stomach and know nothing of our legs, grown tired with sitting. With sexual intercourse it is not that two individuals encased within their bodies place their sexual organ at the disposal of the other, the mere thought might render intercourse impossible; in the sexual intercourse man and woman become sexual organ, their body is transformed into sexual body. A tremendous transformation, of which however anatomist and physiologist will ascertain very little, rather; of *this* transformation they will ascertain nothing. What they ascertain belongs to a very different order of things; to the order of reflective and consequently *gnostic* knowledge, whereas the transformation of the body of the lovers belongs to the order of *"pre-reflective"* and through this in the first place *pathical* experience.

The "pre-reflective" body (which we *are)* therefore has organs, but these organs are far from identical with those of the anatomical and physiological textbooks. It is already a long time that psychoanalytical psychology and psychosomatical medicine have understood that the physical disturbances of the psychiatrical patients cannot be gauged by means of an ordinary medical examination, because such an examination is directed at organs that the patients have not in mind. When a man suffering from an ulcer complains of his stomach, then he does not mean the anatomically definable organ below the diaphragm, but that essentially other organ which receives when a man eats and which digests. Eating must also here be taken "pre-reflectively": as an example of taking in general, of greeting, receiving and welcoming. In the same way that digesting has not here the meaning of a physico-chemical process, but of assimilating in general, of the merging into oneself what everyday life offers, of declaring one's solidarity with events and occurrences. In some way the ulcer patient says "no" to life. It may be that he is unspeakably annoyed with life, he devours himself for exasperation, until there is a hole in his stomach, which also becomes visible in that other organ which the anatomist has in mind. Alexander and French demonstrate in their important publication on *Psychosomatic Medicine* (1948) that it is not possible to sum up the psychopathology of for instance the ulcer patient in one single formula. The above remarks would therefore certainly not profess to universal validity. The point in question is to make it plain that psychopathologist and anatomist do not refer to the same organ *stomach* and that it would be of great value if we succeeded in giving a description of what we refer to under the name of "pre-reflective stomach." Only after this has been achieved may we expect that psychosomatic medicine will not peter out in contradictions. Another example. The patient suffering from *essential hypertension* complains of a feeling of tightness in his head, occasionally in his whole body. He nearly bursts from his vessels, but these are not always in the first place the vessels of the textbook. They are the "pre-reflective vessels," which everybody knows when "the blood flies to his head," when "he blushes," "grows white with anger," or "flushes with hatred or annoyance." They are the vessels whose walls stand for the boundaries of shame or a halt to impulsiveness, the walls with which kept down aggression comes into collision. Shame does not exist as a "purely psychical" quality. Shame is as Mme. Guyon expresses it "that which encompasses the body, encases it like a garment," shame always has a physical meaning, it "is seated" at the boundaries, the walls of the body. *All* so-called "purely psychical qualities" are ways in which the *body* is Hved. The voices of the aggressive people are hard, their muscles are bunched, their blood pulses more fiercely through the vessels. The constantly curtailed, restrained aggression, the aggression which must be kept "within bounds" is a quality of the body as well, a quality to which the name of "hypertension" may be given. This "pre-reflective hypertension" might of course also be registered by the tension meter or ends in a rupture of the anatomically demonstrable vessel. We must enter a note at once also with this example that no attempt is being made here to express hypertension by means of a general and certainly far too easy a psychopathological formula. Our sole intention is to give an illustration of the distinction, but too often neglected, between the body as it is described in the medical textbooks (the body that we *have)* and the body as it plays a part in the non-scientific, not in the first place gnostic, but especially pathi-cal, "pre-reflective" life of man (the body that we *are).*

The patient we described at the beginning of this book does not suffer from psychosomatic disturbances in the strict sense of the word. During an exhaustive physical examination no deviations are found. He "gives a physical expression to a psychical conflict," he *converts.* We can leave the theoretical difficulties of the distinction between psycho-somatical suffering and conversion undiscussed. What these two undoubtedly have in common is that the physical complaint of the patient refers to the "pre-reflective body." Our patient is convinced that his heart is diseased. The internal medicine specialist says that the heart is sound. His information makes curiously little impression on the patient however. We now understand the reason: physician and patient refer to two entirely different organs. The patient speaks of the heart of which it is said that it is "in the right place" or no longer so, whereas the anatomist cannot find even the minutest displacement. The heart that can "leap into my mouth," that can "sink" and that occasionally "is worn on the sleeve," that can be "broken" by words, by a gesture or by a look, whereas the pathologist-anatomist cannot discover any vestige of this terrible rupture. The heart that can be "sound" also when the cardiologist makes a very grave face. And which may very well be "diseased" while all the physicians in the world unanimously declare that the heart they examine functions faultlessly. Whoever speaks of "giving a physical expression to a psychical conflict" really confuses two essentially different things. He who says that the patient *converts* (converto = to change, to transmit, to transmit from one order to another), forgets that the patient does not speak at all of the organs which the physician has in mind, so that he therefore does not trans-mit, not trans-late at all, but remains within the order of one reality, where the scientific distinction between body and soul is not made. The patient's heart *is* ill, he is neither mistaken nor deluded, he has a perfectly real "heartache." For the heart he refers to is the living, beating center of his personal existence, the warm center of a colourful, inspiring world. That the patient is disturbed in this pathical center, that his heart has cooled down, will not be doubted by anyone. His "heart is perturbed," it beats rebelliously in his chest. The patient complains moreover of a weakness in his legs and of feeling as if he would lose his balance. That the neurologist fails to find a deviation need not surprise us now any longer. His reflex hammer does not touch the legs the patient means. It is in a different, much more general sense that "his legs fail him." He can no longer "keep his standing-place in life," his "position is extremely shaky," his "balance" is indeed seriously upset. He threatens to fall, a fall which, if it happens, would also become visible when the legs of the textbook fail him.

The analysis of the physical complaints is not finished. Putting the results of the investigation into the nature of the patient's world by the side of what has just been established, we are struck by a remarkable harmony between them. The patient says that the old and decrepit looking houses are about to tumble down, his world *is* that of the approaching collapse. Must not it strike us that in different words he draws the same picture when he says that his legs fail him and he feels like losing his balance? It is becoming probable that our distinction between *world* and *body* has been too absolute.

As far back as 1935, Buytendijk and Plessner *(Acta Bio-theoretka,* A, I) upheld the view that the physical behavior of man and animal can never be understood if we do not start from the question in what world they live. The authors define the physical behavior as *the answer,* they regard the relationship between body and world as a continuous "conversation," I want to illustrate this in my opinion very important view with a few examples,

A young girl has an evening off. She plans to go into town and she hopes to draw the attention of the young men she will meet. She puts on her best things and makes up her face. When she is ready she examines the result in the glass. Or rather, thus the phenomenologist would reason, she lets, while inspecting herself in the glass, others look through her eyes at "that young girl over there in the glass." If these others "say": "how nice she looks," she gets up and trips for a minute through her room. She *is* then in town already; solely as a result of being already in town she can trip, she can flirt a moment. Then she leaves her room and says goodbye to her parents. Her behavior is entirely different then. She does not trip, she moves like a girl not yet grown up, like a child. There is no need for her parents to criticize her behavior. She "does not restrain herself," there is no question of correction, the change in her behavior is quite "natural." This means: at the moment of her leaving she is so much the child that her behavior must follow suit. Her body responds to the word that the things of her parents' house are still calling out at her: you are a child! As soon as she is in town, another word is addressed to her: the streets glitter with a light she never saw as a child, which stamps her as a grown-up; the looks of the passers-by prove to her that she is dressed as a young woman, that she has a grown-up body. Her body responds: it trips, flirts and is coquettish.

Why is it required of a soldier that his attitude is one of perfect symmetry while reporting himself? Because the meaning of the orders he receives should beforehand be but this: the soldier's world is not that of "possibly," of "perhaps," "perhaps not," in this world everything has its own fixed place, the aims are well denned and are to be attained by no roundabout ways. Why has within living memory the attitude of him who prays been preferably symmetrical? Because the world of him who prays, though differing from that of the soldier, is given a definite direction, a direction without any qualifications, without any prevarications. For the moment the praying man expels all dubiousness from the things of his existence. Why is the attitude of the adolescent so strikingly asymmetrical? Because in his world nothing has as yet a fixed place, everything is "askew," all is dubious and every direction suggests numerous roundabout ways. The body, says Von Gebsattel* *moulds itself* in dose resemblance to the plan of the world in which it finds its task sketched out, it assumes a shape, a *form:* a work er's form in response to the invitation issuing from a workshop, a warrior's form in response to the appeal of an arena, a lover's form in response to the erotic approach of the beloved. The prereflective body and the prereflective world are engaged in a continuous dialogue. Both can only be understood from this dialogue.

In his article on experiencing space *(Nervertarzt,* V, 1930), Erwin Straus shows us an excellent psychiatric example. The author asks himself in what way it must be psychologically understood that the catatonic is motionless. He formulates the answer by pointing to the fact that the catatonic lives in a space quite different from ours. Our healthy space is characterized by direction, usefulness, aim and intention. The motor bus that I see standing at the stopping-place is for me at once a conveyance going from . . . to . . . , even though I don't know the names of the starting-point and the terminus. It has an intention, a direction, usefulness. That is how I see it. The flowers in the living-room I see at once as a decoration of this space, I see them at the same time as just opening their buds," my seeing measures the time they will remain, fresh. The catatonic no doubt sees quite otherwise. It is well known that on being asked in what year he was born, he often mentions the year when his psychosis began, since then he "did not grow any older," time does not flow any longer. Consequently he does not see flowers "opening their buds," nor a motor bus from, to. Neither does he see use or intention. We ask him in vain why the flowers stand in the living-room. He makes no answer to the question what is the use of the bus. Every change or removal of things is senseless to him, opaque, superfluous, better still: impossible. All things have become rigid in a timeless space. The body responds to this by not moving any more. The catatonic stands like a statue in a museum of curiosities. Whereas to us, non-cata.tonics, the world so dearly world is agitated, i.e., when to our mind all things vibrate, when everywhere there is violent turbulence and rapid change, then we ourselves are also hurried. "Has" the world "time," i.e., when the things of life speak to us of rest, perhaps even convey at times the eternity idea of creation, then our movements slow down too. The townsman moves in a rush, the peasant moves soberly, there is something of solemnity in the slow step of the monk and in the movement of his hand.

For the *melancholiac* the stream of life moves sluggishly, he sees the laborious movement of every change, therefore his movements are heavy and slow; the aspect of the world is colorless, spiritless and faded, therefore he feels tired, spent, weary and dull. For the *maniac* visible life goes lightly, obstacles there are none, his movements are correspondingly quick and light; the world is all life and movement, full of brilliant hues and freshness, that is why he himself feels fresh and alive, he feels so light that in this world, from which all weight has been taken away, he could almost fly (Binswanger). The incipient *schizophrenic* sees himself surrounded by unmistakable indications of the destruction of the world. He scents hell, he discerns the ruinous work of diabolical forces. Can we wonder that he complains that his body is at the mercy of occult powers? "They" cut off his thoughts, "they" belabour him with infernal machinery. His body responds to the physiognomy of an infernal world.

Indeed, the distinction between body and world is considerably less hard and fast than we, under the influence of Cartesian trains of thought, are usually led to think! We shall learn from the next paragraph that a number of other distinctions are as a rule also taken far too rigorously.

3. MAN AND FELLOW MAN. COMMUNICATION

ID his autobiography 5; *le grain me meurt* the French writer Andre Gide describes an occurrence from his youth which, in my opinion, throws a remarkable light on the nature of inter-

indicates movement, so very visibly is "in motion" that we cannot but respond to this appeal by movements of our body. When the human contact. He tells of a walk which as a child he took with his nurse. It was, so the story runs, in the middle of summer and the two of them were picking flowers in a valley not far from their holiday residence. In order to ascertain that the girl had not wandered too far away from him he glanced up. In that very moment she emerged from the deep shade under an ashtree into the full sunlight. In her hand she held a bunch of marsh spiraeas, she wore a light summer hat, whose broad brim protected her face from the sun. She seemed to him, as she laughed, to be summer itself. He asked what it was that made her laugh: "Why are you laughing?" She answered gaily: "Because I am! It is such lovely weather!" At that moment, says Gide, *the valley was fitted with love and happiness.*

This simple example, which everyone is sure to recognize, because in some connection or other he will have had the same experience, shows us that a word spoken by a person we love, can throw an entirely new and unexpected glow over the world —in this case over a valley. It may be that I am too hasty, I may expect that several psychologists wish to enter a protest against this seemingly too facile conclusion. It was not the words of the nurse that had changed the valley, they will protest, but these words delighted young Gide and after that he projected his joy in the valley. The valley after all had not changed its aspect, it had "on closer inspection" remained exactly the same, the sunlight had not become more summery nor have the colors of the flowers deepened. The phenomenol-ogist in his turn will now enter a protest. In the first place he will remark that "on closer inspection" is not the way in which a psychologist ought to look at things, since "on closer inspection" reduces everything to that which can be observed "in cold blood," whereas the daily living observation rarely takes place "in cold blood" and as a result sees quite other things. Whoever wishes to know what happens psychologically, does well *to enter - fully into the situation,* he should be careful as an outsider not to pass judgment too easily *on* the situation. Who enters into Gide's situation *sees* with him a new valley, where the sunlight is indeed more summer-like and where the colors of the flowers really are more brilliant.—In the second place the phenomenologist will observe that Gide makes no mention of any joy that first had only been his and afterwards became visible in the landscape. He does not breathe a word of any free interval, during which something like a projection took place. Who supposes that this free interval was too short to be noticed, would certainly have been told by Gide that should there have been any question of an interval, he would have expected this interval *after* rather than *before* the transformation of the valley: the change of the valley, the visible flooding "with love and with joy" made him glad; it was not his joy that gave greater beauty to the valley.—We should stick to the facts! For could it ever be the intention of psychology to distort the facts for the sake of a fine theory? For this must be said: who would explain Gide's experience by means of the projection theory does violence to the facts. We have paid sufficient attention to all this in the previous pages.

Keeping to Gide's experience we must say: the words, the exclamation of the nurse filled the world with a new glow.

We noted already that Gide was on excellent terms with the nurse. It is not so much a question of the word that is uttered, it is a question of the person who reveals himself in the words. Or rather: it is the tie between two people that endows the word with special power. A power for the good or a power for the bad. For let us suppose that Gide hated his nurse. The rest of the scene may remain the same, indeed the words uttered by the girl might have been identical, the effect of these words would no doubt have been a darkening of the valley. Ten to one the sun would have burned hard and pitilessly and the hues of the flowers would have acquired a fairly poisonous aspect. In a Dutch novel treating of a marriage that went wrong (De verborgen bron *[The Hidden Source}* by Hella. Haasse) the man writes a letter to his wife about his experiences during a visit to a house left to him as a legacy. He is enthusiastic about what he saw and in his delight he writes: "I wish you were here!" Then he apparently remembers how deep a chasm sep- arates them and continues: "I *don't* wish it after all, probably because 1 should be afraid that I should see with your eyes then," Let us suppose that he had not made this correction and that she, at his request had travelled to where he was and had wandered together with him through the house that so greatly roused his delight. If we believe the author, in that case he would see the house *with other eyes,* that is, -*with her eyes* (_the phenomenologist takes this literally). "While she was looking at it with him, the house would have taken on another aspect, less inviting, less desirable, less habitable. We have every reason to believe the author. Everyone knows persons with whom he would not by preference see a town, a museum or a landscape, because he wishes to leave the aspect of the things to be found there unspoilt. Just as everyone knows people with whom a walk in a town or in the country adds new, unknown and excellent aspects to what we behold. The lattet we call our friends, our beloved, our husband or wife. In his publication, inexhaustible for the psychologist *(A la recherche du temps perdu)*, Marcel Proust relates how as a young man, during a walk, he once felt a burning wish to be with a girl. As soon as this wish arose the appearance of the landscape changed. Her imagined presence added a "new quality to the landscape." He sees this addition "in the colour of the tiles on the farms, in the herbs growing around him," it Hes "on the village dreaming in the distance." What he sees is but his awakening love, he perceives the tie with the imagined girl. Together with her he would have liked to walk, to talk and to look.

Let us summarize as follows. The word, the look or the gesture of a fellow man can brighten or darken my world. The fellow man is not another isolated entity, standing beside me, pouring words into my ear; who, just as myself, would remain foreign to the things of the world. He is primarily one who is or is not "together" with me and the degree of this being together with me or not is no metaphysical abstraction, but a reality, visible in the things which he and I observe. Our being together or not appears in the physiognomy of the world. The physiognomy may be familiar or unfamiliar, near or far. The being together with a fellow man interprets itself into a nearness to or a distance from the observable. The word of the nurse (with whom Gide was on excellent terms) renders the valley surprisingly "near." The eye of the wife (between whom and the man the married relationship was not a happy one) would have moved the house to a disappointing "distance."

That a fellow man very often increases the distance between myself and my world (or my task, the task always being a more or less inviting, in some cases perhaps compelling aspect of the world) is strikingly illustrated by the French existentialist Jean-Paul Sartre. Here follows an example. A man looks through the keyhole into a room where incidents occur not meant for his eyes. He is quite absorbed in what he sees. The scene is very "near" to him, he has, so to say, crept through the keyhole (the phenomenologist is inclined to take this fairly literally) and has left his body standing outside the door: that this body in its awkward position is getting tired does not occur to him, so completely is he "with" the incidents. Until he hears footsteps behind him. Before he can straighten himself the room beyond the door is taken away from him. What was near becomes, owing to the presence behind his back, all at once very far away. This distance remains when he discovers that the other decidedly disapproves of his conduct. It might be however that the other is the same person together with whom he had already more than once looked through that keyhole before. Immediately the enclosed spectacle is near again and it is quite likely, owing to the other's taking an eager share in the observation, to come even nearer and to grow at the same time more interesting and more piquant.

We had planned in this paragraph to answer the question what the position is of the relationship of man and man. The answer has seemingly led us rather far away from the question. Instead of telling something further and making things clearer regarding the tie existing "between" people, the answer points to the world being far or near. It is simple enough to trace the cause of this curious shifting. Until a short time ago psychology rested on that philosophical interpretation of man regarding him as a subject enclosed in the body, unable to have any original contact with the things of the world. The world was foreign to him, it would only in a certain sense become his when he sprayed his libido over it. Or rather: it would never really belong to him, for what he regarded as the intimaq- of things always ultimately belonged to his strictly subjective property. The world was not important. It is in absolute accord with this interpretation that they expected mutual human contact to be found in a tie existing *between* them. Psychology remained uneasily conscious however of the fact that there was never anything really satisfactory to be said about this *between*. The extensive literature about the "Einfiihlen" serves as a fascinating illustration. Phenomenological psychology on the contrary holds in memory that there is an original contact of man with things. The cobbler "forgets" himself, he is lost in his work, he "becomes" the shoe that is to be repaired. The novelist "becomes" his novel (if his work is to be good), the mathematician "becomes" his problem, he enters into this problem, he liberates himself when he carries his problem to a good conclusion. Once it has been realized that the rigorous separation of man and world rests on a philosophical prejudice and that no justice is done to the reality of man and world, we will be on our guard against trying to find the contact of man with man in a tie which would exist "between" two worldless subjects. From this reflection results our answer: the relationship of man with man is embodied in the physiognomy of things, in the world's being far or near.

Still this answer cannot possibly be complete. For there is also another kind of human contact. We shake hands with a person, we put a friendly hand on a person's shoulder, or warningly tap his arm. We look at each other, we look into each other's eyes, we can even in a way "sink" our eyes into another's. The amorous couple link their little fingers, their hands; they link arms. There is an embracing, an entwining of two bodies, a kiss, caresses, sexual intercourse. Nobody would uphold the view—an occasional attempt has been made—that it is here only a question of a contact of two factually anonymous bodies. The touch is a contact of one human being with another, direct, without any shield in between, an immediate participating in each other, A handshake for instance can para-digmatically reveal to me the nature of the contact. Everyone knows the handshake that amounts to a belittlement, a revile-ment or an insult. There exists besides a whole category of handshakes revealing the nearness of the other, his friendship or love, ^e speak of a cold, a cool, a warm and even of a heated handshake, their temperatures being the temperatures of the contact itself of man with man, they have conveyed themselves to the handshakes, these temperatures, they are registered and the registered height is the nature of the contact. The temperature of a handshake! One is well advised to leave the thermometer at home when taking these temperatures. Here we again encounter the distinction already mentioned a few times of two kinds of observation: the direct, "psychological" observation and that "on closer inspection." The latter, which until recently enjoyed undisputed hegemony in psychology, would observe *nothing* from that handshake, whereas in daily life the differences in temperature of the handshake are entitled to indisputable reality. Let us give some further illustration. Everyone knows the handshake of the arrogant man, the "condescending" handshake, the hand "like a dead fish." This hand is to the immediate "pre~reflective" perception of him who re-ceives it long, narrow and chilly, the fingers *are* thin. Yet it might very well be the case that an objective measuring, i.e., an observation "on closer inspection" yields very different results. The hand may turn out not to be long and narrow at all, but on the contrary comparatively short and thick. The thermometer might in this case also show us that the hand is fairly warm, etc. The psychologist who wants to put his trust exclusively in the objective observation, simply crosses off the chapter about the handshake.

Phenomenology is a science of examples. Driven by the need to keep as closely as possible to the events of daily life (in the form in which these events actually occur) it develops by going from one example to another. The example that can serve us for the closer studying of the nature of physical contact is borrowed from Sartre's chief work *L'etre et le neanf.*

When I look at the back of my hanH, says Sartre, I discover veins that form a very definite configuration. These configurations are different for the left and the right hand

and when I look at other people's hands it becomes apparent that there are no two hands to be found showing a perfectly identical configuration of the veins. The situation is the same as that of the finger prints; no two persons in the world show an identical picture of the delicate grooves of, for instance, their right hand thumb. There is, Sartre continues, something unsatisfactory about this discovery, it gives me a curious feeling of dissatisfaction. Of course the veins in the back of my hand must have a certain course: they are there, they are necessary, they must be somewhere. But why do they lie just there where I see them, why is their course in my right hand different from that in my left hand and why is their arrangement in ray hand different from that of any other person I meet? They evidently serve their purpose just as well when they run differently. Why then do they lie just there? Nobody will be able to answer this question at all satisfactorily. All the same, Sartre says, I know the situation when my dissatisfaction suddenly flies. As soon as a person, a woman who loves me and whom I love, caresses my hand, I become convinced that the veins tun exactly as they should. The caress cancels the accidentalitv of my hand, it turns it into "exactly that hand which it should be fit for me to have."

It is in the caress that a profound transformation of the body takes place (a transformation of which the physiologist perceives nothing). As an individual I always feel more or less strange to my body. I see that it has a certain shape, not particularly desired nor undesiied either, and that it, equally without my will being concerned, possesses very definite characteristics of behavior. I have to accept the shape and the qualities much as I should have to accept the uncertainties of a climate, I go on regarding them with a certain suspicion. Until somebody else teaches me that I may also *be* this body that I *have,* may exactly be it as it is. In the caress the accidentality of the body is removed, there takes place a justification of my body; the caress wipes out the distance between myself and my body, there occurs an adhesion of myself and my body, I begin to inhabit this body, I am invited *to be* this body.

One's fellow man plays a part in the relationship of man and his body. He may make this relationship closer. On the other hand he may also make it more remote, he may increase the distance between my body and myself. There can be found an enormous number of cases in point. The freckled girl continuously lives on a hostile footing with her body, because she never forgets that others ridicule these freckles. The poor valuation of these others forms a barrier between her and her body. Until a young man tells her or in another way convincingly proves to her that he loves her as she is, freckles and all.

Perhaps he loves her for this very reason, because she has freckles and so many more things that other girls are without. For this is the peculiarity of love: it arises from the particularities the beloved possesses, particularities not found anywhere except in her. The special, exceptional qualities which usually form that which, owing to the opinion of "the others" is the cause of the bad footing on which one is with one's body, yet may apparently be the first motive for love.

In a preceding paragraph we spoke of a man who is spying through the keyhole into a room not meant for his eyes.

At the moment he hears the footsteps behind him he is deprived of the spectacle. But there happens something else as well, A tremendous difference is effected simultaneously between him and his body. He imitates the disapproving look of the other, he sees his own body *through the other's eyes* (the phenomenologist takes this literally) and like the other he criticizes that body over there.

The word, the gesture and the look of a fellow man may increase or lessen the distance between man and his body, they may render the body (just as the world) less or more habitable, —That a singular mixture of this less and this more may sometimes occur may be seen from the fin^l example,

A girl of about 16 enters the room where her elder brother sits talking with a couple of friends. When they see who is coming in, they stop talking for a moment and look at her. For the first time in her life the girl perceives that she is regarded by male eyes. She blushes. What is the meaning of this blushing? There is a great difference in the way in which a man looks and a woman. Whereas the eye of a woman predominantly *rests* on things and people, a man usually looks straight through things, his look wants to fathom, to unmask, to change (Buytendijk, *De vrottw,* 1951). The girl perceives that she is regarded with this look; her brother's friends regard her with this unmasking look, they look through her clothes, their eyes divine from the neck the breast, from the ankle the thigh, their eyes try to unclothe her. Her body is taken from her, it has turned object to the friends of her brother. But things do not stop at this disheartening estrangement from her own body. For the first time in her life too she feels within het the wish to inhabit this new body, made new that is by the others. Under these looks she turns into a woman. She wants *to be* this new body and to prove this her body is flooded with blood; it becomes visible, stitt more visible than it had become already under the eyes of the young men. She is entering this body with her blood. But her shame is at the same time a barrier to hide behind, a barrier against the male eye piercing all; her blush as distinctly says no. Her blush is the resultant of her estrangement from her body *and* a new intimacy of her body. The other's look rendered her body simultaneously inhabitable and uninhabitable.

We can now formulate the phenomenological answer to the question what the situation is regarding the relationship of man with man. *The relation of man with man becomes real in the physiognomy, the vicinity or the distance, of world and body.*

The right thing to do would seem to me to finally illustrate this definition with the psychology of an ordinary conversation. My friend and I are talking together. This talking "together" always means that we talk about "something." We are speaking of Iceland, where we have never been, but which we slightly know from books. We are not speaking of "the picture we have formed of Iceland," no: we mean Iceland as it is, we are speaking of the world. While my friend is discussing it, I try to enter into what he says. However wrong our ideas may be, I try to "enter into" this Iceland, lying at hand. And while I talk, he tries to enter into what I tell him. This "trying to enter" *is* our friendship. For, if I were speaking with a dis agreeable person, then our words, even if they were the identical ones of the talk with my friend, would not be "a trying to enter into" and this "not trying or not wishing to enter" would be our antipathy. In the talk with my friend I "see" Iceland, as it is taking shape in our words. But at the same time I see him and he sees me. I see his enthusiastic look with which he is regarding Iceland. I let my eyes glance for an instant over the face whose expression harmonizes with that Iceland over there, which he is calling up for me. I see his whole body at a glance. And I appreciate his look, his face, his body, an appreciation of which my friend is conscious, however vague and implicit it is. My appreciation sets him free to speak as he does, to look so enthusiastically, to move his body and shape it as he does. My presence is no critique on his way of expression, but a justification of this way. Under my regard his body may be such as this body is when it speaks. My speaking, hearing and seeing with him and my seeing his speaking body effects an adhesion of him and his body. This adhesion then is nothing but the tie "between" him and myself: our friendship.

With me it is no different. Speaking about that Iceland yonder which I *see* (I see no *picture,* my imagining means the country lying in the north of the Atlantic Ocean; the supposition that the imagining is directed at a picture, not at reality, is also the product of a psychology that separates man from his world), I enter with great freedom "into that Iceland," I dare go and "live in it," because the friendship with my friend has removed the barrier between myself and the world. The absence of the barrier is the friendship existing "between" him and me*. And at the same time I know that he regards me, he sees me gesticulate, talk and look. I move my body with the same freedom, without any obstruction I flow into my arms, my hands, into my throat and mouth, into my eyes. I go and inhabit my body and that I can inhabit my body only means that I am on good terms with my friend.

In the paragraph treating tie relationship of man and body it was seen that the separation of body and world should by no means be regarded as too rigorous. Body and world are engaged in a dialogue. The wodd invites the body to assume a certain shape, the body ia answer to this invitation forms itself. In agreement with thb the changes of the world and the body, as these take place for instance in conversation, are not two occurrences happening independently of one another. The response of our bodies to the fact that my friend and I in our conversation inhabit Iceland is an inhabitableness becoming greater in proportion.

A few more words now about the patient in Chapter I. He says that the things around him have become alien, he cannot inhabit these things any more. This means already that he has no proper contact with people. He goes on to say that his body has changed, he has no confidence in this body any more, he is afraid that his heart, this centre of his physical existence will fail. In saying so he tells us for the second time that he is on bad terms with people; his fellow men will be to him an insurmountable barrier, preventing him to freely inhabit his body, just as these fellow men act as impassable obstacles in the matter of a truly human habitation of his world. If moreover he also tells us that people appear to him as hostile, rigid puppets, then in different words he once more gives expression to what is his real disturbance, about which he wants to consult the psychotherapist: he is very seriously disturbed in the contact with others. For the deepest sense of our existence is lodged within our fellow men. If we can really see a *smile* in his smile then the world sparkles with forms, colors and light, our body stands erect, our look is free. If we see his smile as a sneer, then things wilt and molder around us, all color fades and light becomes a faint glimmer; our body also decays.

What we are very anxious to know now is how the patient drifted into such a disturbance. What is it that happened in his life which was the cause that nearly everybody is his enemy? What is the origin of his serious neurosis?

In the following paragraph we shall try to find an answer to this question. In this connection it will be necessary first to come to understand the relation of man and his *time*.

4. MAN AND TIME. LIFE HISTORY

In his *Con-fessiones* (XI, 14) St. Augustine asks a question, probably the most difficult that a man can ever ask himself. He asks "what is time?" and as soon as he makes an attempt to formulate an answer he gets into a curious quandary. "When no one asks me what time is," so he says, "I know, but when I would give an explanation of it in answer to a man's question I do not know." Time is a matter of course in our daily life. Unhesitatingly we take out our watch to see the time, we unerringly localize an event that happened long ago, we make appointments for the days ahead, we dearly realize the flowing of time, even when we have been asleep, we usually know that time has passed, we ascertain that time moves quickly or slowly —should we want however to know what time is, *what* it is that flows and how this flowing must be imagined, then we seek in vain for an even slightly acceptable explanation. This is not only true for time, the same lament might be heard when asking ourselves the question: what is space? or; what is our body? or: what after all is contact between men? None of all these questions harass us in ordinary daily life or anyhow only very little: we take possession of space, travel, fly, go in somewhere or come out; we use our body as if we are it ourselves (as we usually are), we move, bathe or lie in the sun; without thinking about it we hold out a hand to a person, we talk together, get married. One would almost say: we *live* the answers to all these questions without any problems arising worth mentioning, but if we stop to think about it, if we try to submit these questions to reflection, then there are incalculable difficulties. What is clear*((pre-reflectively"* becomes obscure *reflectively*. Now phenomenology is that remarkable science, audaciously making the pretence, too audaciously in the opinion no doubt of some, to try and find the answer to these questions not reflectively this time but "pre-reflectively."

Too audaciously, for how is one to think, to reflect about that which, when defined, proves to take place before and beyond all reflection? This seems a glaring impossibility.

Naturally the phenomenologist sees this difficulty dearly. But he will not say that this difficulty implies an impossibility. In order to arrive at an exposition of the prereflective, he will say, I will quite decidedly turn away from the usual method of thinking. Instead of giving expression to an always reflective and. as the history of thought teaches us never satisfying *theory of* the problems given, I will let the problem speak for itself. In the preceding pages we have discussed some examples already. When the question was asked as to the situation of the relationship of man and world, we started from the simplest possible example: that of the man and the bottle of wine and we gave the winebottle, i.e., the place where in this case the relation of man and world materializes, *the opportunity to speak.* Quite true, we let ourselves say what the winebottle tells us and our story intended to be as true a copy as possible of the story that we heard.

Things speak to us, we know—the poet for instance and the painter know this so very well, that is why poets and painters are born phenomenologists—it may even be assumed that by virtue of this being spoken to we handle things so unerringly; that by virtue of our understanding this remarkable language of things, we continually *live* a solution of the problems which, to reflection prove to be so hopelessly unsolvable. The farmer grasps the plough because the plough asks him to be thus grasped, he ploughs the earth because the earth calls for this action. The swimmer entrusts himself to the water because the water tells him in a thousand different ways that it will receive his body kindly. We decide to go and live in a house because already during the viewing the rooms began to tell us of what is going to happen there in the future: it tells us of the home coming there, of its warmth in winter, of freshness there in summer etc.

Phenomenology is before everything a methodical adjustment, an *attitude* as it were. Its method is a new way of observing, new in science, new for instance in psychology, but in no way new to man in general. On the contrary: the phenomenologist wants to observe as man *usually* observes. He has a great and unshaken confidence in the usual way of observing things, the body, his fellow men, also of time for this reason that *this observing brings about the solution of the problems.* He has a profound distrust of the theoretical observation, the observing "objectively," the observing "on closer inspection," that manner of observation which in an extreme form bears such good fruit to the physicist. He distrusts judgment equally profoundly, too easy judgments, such as: projection, conversion, transference and sublimation. He is convinced that these and similar judgments span "pre-reflective" clarity with a *theory,* an easy one, but not for this reason correct, and as a rule also very foggy. He wants to postpone judgment to the last moment and before all to listen to what events, life, in short the *phenomena* have to *say* to him (phenomeno-logy). And his narrative means to be no more than the truest possible report of what he observes, hears, sees, smells, and feels.

He wants to live himself and from this life to make his psychology to come forth. Planning to write a treatise on swimming, he will first go and swim; only he who knows the sea, the river, the brook and the lake personally, i.e., with his body, will be able to say something about swimming. He can make the water speak to him and his body responds, the psychology of swimming is nothing but a faithful report of this dialogue. If he wants to know something more about interhuman contact, he will go and move among people and carefully be on his guard against hatching out some sterile theory in his study.

All this sounds too easy, of course. The phenomenologist is quite conscious of the fact that he—however much he would desire otherwise—often turns away to what is theoretical, consequently foreign to life. He also knows that pre-phenomeno-logkal psychology yielded splendid results.

Let as now see how the phenomenologist approaches the question *"what is time"* and what he can observe during this approach. True to his method, he starts with the description of a simple and inconspicuous incident.

One day a psychically healthy young man happened to be talking with his parents about events in his youth. "What will remain with me through life," he said smiling, "are the Sunday afternoons. I believe the feeling is still there, that every Sunday afternoon is tainted by the memory of those early days. What a bore they were!" On his parents asking him what memory he meant, he said: "Well, surely, you must remember. We never were so rebellious and refractory as when father had finished his afternoon nap and you said: 'Now we are going for our walk!' We were dressed in our best suits, our new boots were put on and we departed, duly warned not to walk on the damp grass, not to step in the mud, to say nothing of climbing trees and such like. We used to encounter some other parents with children equally finely dressed, looking equally blue. The four grown-ups embarked on a conversation, which lasted endlessly and we bad to keep hanging around." "How often do you think this happened?" asked his parents amused. "Oh well, I can't remember exactly of course, but at a guess I should say every other Sunday at least." "You are very greatly mistaken then," his parents replied, "we did not relish such 'proper' walks ourselves at all on Sunday afternoons. But now and then there was no avoiding them: we had to make calls occasionally. It will have happened no oftener than once in three months. And as to those conversations in the street, we exchanged a couple of words and continued our way after two or three minutes."

There is no need to be a neurotic in order to "mythify" the past. On the contrary, this "mythification" is the rule with the healthy as well as with the sick. Nobody returns to the place where he lived in his early youth in after years without being in some way disappointed: it used to be different, more intimate, says the man in good health; more wretched, says the neurotic. The proportions of the houses, their doors, their windows, the size and aspect of the streets, the lights going up in those streets in the evening, the early morning sounds, the summery character of the summers, the wintery character of the winters: it all used to be "different," and it is this "different," which on our return cannot be verified, that we allow to determine our present life, even the future. The aforementioned young man will know better than to try to induce his own children to come for a walk on Sunday afternoons in later years. His memory, not shared at all by his parents, determines the way in which he educates his children.

The first thing we must say of the *past,* when we let this past speak to us, is that it affects us as a sound, operative in *the present.* The chief importance of the past does not lie in the time in which it was enacted, it may be of very slight importance there, the past speaks in our present-day existence. There were innumerable Sunday afternoons spent in complete freedom: that was the value of the past when it was actual. The past that is being lived, which is significant for him who has to live with this past, is the past *as if appears m the present.* The past is, if we would express it thus, a *presentatjve* past.

One of my acquaintances told me that after the war she visited the prison where she had had to spend a very anxious time during the occupation. Her comparative composure at the arrest had soon fled, when during the interrogations she found out what they accused her of and in what way the accusations were formulated. What struck her so extraordinarily at her visit after the war was that the prison door proved to be so much smaller than she had imagined. "I had pictured the door at least twice as high and twice as wide," she said. When I asked her what she thought of the size of the door now, she said smiling "well, to tell you the truth, it really was an enormous door I passed, I think so still!" Of course she knew that the door that had closed behind her a few years before, was the objectively controllable size that had struck her when she paid her carefree visit. But this size did not belong to the past with which she had to count when remembering the occupation period. In the past which had her in its grasp, this door remained large: the enormous door that closed on liberty. We must even say that, immediately after the war, she had a perfect right to remember this door as a very large one. The discrepancy between war and peace, occupation and liberty, foreign domination and self determination was still at that time so bumingly real, that the prison door, just as so many other things in her life, needs must appear to her in this "burning" guise. The fad: is that what concerns us never exists as what is called "conscious state," but confronts us in the physiognomy of things. At the liberation bread was whiter than ever before and nobody will succeed in taking the conviction from me that bread never was so white and—let us hope—will never be so white again. The airplanes bringing the first food and flying low over the city of Utrecht never had such a heavy cargo and never had such a gravely benevolent flight as then and I shall never suffer this impression to be taken away from me, even though I am told that the present-day planes can carry three or four times that weight. The present-day guise in which the past appears to me has a part to play. As long as this part has not been accomplished, this past—all objective control notwithstanding—will speak to me in the same voice. The proportions of the prison door can certainly become reduced, but not by using a yardstick. We can imagine that the prisoner of those days through frequent contacts with the enemy of those days can take away from that enemy the odium of hostility. Should this happen, then the part of the "big door" will be played out, The door has then become an "ordinary door" again. As to the Sunday afternoons, the young man does not by means of this memory demonstrate the frailty of human remembrance, he demonstrates that the education given by his parents was no empty thing to him—education never is—it may be that by means of his memory he shows a fragment of immaturity; it is even very well possible that by bringing up this memory during the chat with his parents, he tries to rid himself of this remnant of immaturity. Who after years of absence visits the scene of his early youth and perceives that his memory speaks in far kinder and more intimate words than what he now sees, ascertains that the past has a present value, which is right and which he may preserve. He will say "I had better not come back here" and he is right: it is a good thing that the past will go on speaking to him as it evidently does. The neurotic on the other hand is not right if he does not wish to revisit this scene of his boyhood: he *f.ies* from a present guise of the past, which injures him all the time, it is perhaps the highest time for him to get on a better footing with this past, which always means this: that his memories begin to speak to him so as not to disquiet him$_s$ but to soothe, perhaps to set him free, perhaps, who knows, even to inspire him.

Let us summarize it all as follows. Remembering is not a more or less successfully returning to the anchorage of the more or less happily anchored *engram*. The past is that which was *as it now appears to us*. That which was: certain Sunday afternoons no doubt really consisted in a "proper" walk, but this is the bare skeleton, which will have to be embodied in flesh and blood, if it is to live. And the past does live, it is living *now*. Nor is it without signification that it lives *now* and *in the way* it appears to live. The past plays an actual part, it has to fulfill a mission for the good or for the bad.

It must strike anyone how very little psychology speaks of the *future*. "Whereas we may state that man thinks incomparably more of what is to come than of what has been, that as a rule he Hves in the future, goes to meet the future and comparatively seldom returns to the past, psychology is much more at home in the past than in the future. Is there with the psychologist a certain distrust towards the future? We might begin to suspect this, if we remember the violent controversy between Freud and A. Maeder, when the latter made a cautious attempt to attribute to the dream the signification of an experimental action. The dream performs symbolically what is about to happen. Maeder argued, the dream is not only the product of the —not quite successful—past, it may also be a pointer to what is coming. Freud rejected this with a firmness which makes us suspect that vety fundamental convictions came into play f*Internationale Psycboanalytische und Psychoptttbologische For-scbungen*. Band V, 1913, p. 647). This was in 1913, in the opening period of the psychoanalytical movement, when the doctrine of the psychotraumata as the originators of neurosis celebrated its triumphs. The neurotic had been wrongly brought up, it was only necessary to listen to his reports to know how wretchedly he had been brought up. His neurosis was the result of the deplorable facts of his youth. In those days the psychoanalyst still thought fairly physiologically. These facts were stored as *engrammaia,* these *engrammatet* carry out their destructive work associatively. Everything appeared dear, one would almost say. anatomically clear. Who is still so tied up with physiological trains of thought does not take kindly to assign ing a psychological reality to the future. For there are no *engrammata:* nothing has happened yet, so nothing can have been anchored yet.

The appeal to the future is an appeal to the uncertain, the nebulous. There is not anything to go upon. That we should consider the future does not signify much more than that we lengthen the series of *engrammafa* from long ago up till now by means of a jumping-board to the entirely problematical. The future was not much more than this jumping-board.

We are obliged to say that this picture does not correspond with the reality of our life, and not even with the reality of neurotic life. He who listens intently to those patients cannot but conclude that they undoubtedly let their thoughts go out to what is coming. One even gains the impression that the reason why they are so singularly occupied with the past is that the future appears to them as a muddle of approaching failures and therefore never leaves them alone. They are, like the healthy, in the first place "in the future," but every step they advance in it stirs up a hopelessly entangled past. If it did not sound so queer one would be inclined to say: the past comes to meet them from the future. Or is this not so very strange after all? We shall leave this question for a moment. A simple example is now called for, which we can ask what it is all about, this dark, dim, isolated entity that bears the name of *future*.

I wake up in the morning. Before getting out of bed I allow myself to be taken hold of by the thought of what the day will bring. It does not take much time. The evening before, the day before or perhaps much longer ago already I had made plans for this day or plans were dictated to me by circumstances. I step into the day, which assumed a certain character. Then and there it is clear to me that the way I put my legs out of bed corresponds with the character the day has assumed. There are days that make me get out in a flash, others when it takes a moment for the second leg to follow the first and I even know days whose aspect is so unattractive that I turn over again and pretend that the day has not begun at all. It is evident from this example that the future cannot actually be so vague and isolated an entity as has sometimes been assumed. On the contrary the future seems very real to me, so real that I let myself be entirely determined by it. But how is this possible? How is it possible that I can let my behaviour be determined by "what is coming later," what in no way now already *is*? How can that which is not (yet) in existence influence me?

Speaking thus we start after all from the idea that the future is absolutely what comes *later,* i.e., what must be considered to be quite apart from to-day. But is this right? Is this in conformity with the real facts? Is not it much more correct to say that the present and the future are not so rigorously separated as the clock would tell me, but that a very close tie is likely to exist between the present and the future, so close that we may say that the future lies *contained* in the present, that the future, it is true, is what is later, but *a "later' as it appears to me now?* For, getting out of bed I don't let myself be determined by what is going to happen later in the day; such a thing is indeed •unimaginable; what is really happening later in the day is not yet there and therefore, because it does not exist, can have no influence either. Moreover it is very well possible that what does happen later in the day does not at all accord with the way I move my legs out of bed. The day may happen to pass extremely pleasantly for instance, though I left my bed in the morning in the most unwilling fashion.

The future is: *that which comes, as it comes to meet me now,* The future is *"to-come."* The German speaks of *Zu-kunft,* the Frenchman of *a-venir.* This means: the future is most essentially that which finds expression in the way it comes to meet me. Thinking of the future I am already in what comes hastening towards me. Before I put my legs outside the bed, the day has already come to meet me, I was in the day already before the day began, before I move my legs out of bed and move into the room, I already entered the day. The way of my entering-the-day and the way in which the day hastens to meet me correspond like question and answer, and the fruit of this dialogue is my way of leaving the bed as I do and not as I don't.

Erwin Straus has analyzed all this in an exemplary manner in his excellent book *Vom Smn der Sinne* (1935). His analysis amounts to this. When I leap a ditch, my leap is only comprehensible if the "coming down on the other side" has taken on a form before I leap. He who leaps tests the other bank beforehand, he must come down before he leaps, he can only leap because the future arrival at the other side has acquired a sharply outlined, *actual* form. Before I jump *I am already on the other side* and the way in which I "already am" on the other side determines my leap.

No one goes to swim in a river without his being in one way or another "already in the river" before his foot touches the water. That one person "is already there" in an eager way and another very hesitatingly is proved by the way they set about it. The former takes a flying leap into the water, which he could inhabit so well already before his jump, the latter moves very slowly and with noticeable fear or reluctance into this element, which was to him, already beforehand a cold or a dangerous place. Nobody travels to a country, even though it may be totally unknown to him, without his being "in the country" already at the moment when his journey begins. Trie future always has the somewhat paradoxical meaning of *encountering oneself.* I "was already" in that country; now that I am crossing it by train I encounter myself as it were, I encounter that self which I put down in that country before crossing it by train or on foot. The swimmer who enters the water with so much fear and reluctance probably has every reason for doing so: it will be his earlier experiences, the stories he heard about swimming and drowning, which were the cause that he "is already in such a way in the water" that his real going down into the river can only take place hesitatingly and fearfully.

The past comes to meet him from the future. When the neurotic wants to pay a call and greatly shrinks from the conversation, he puts his experiences of the contacts with others into the future conversation: in this future his past comes to meet him and it may be that his past speaks so convincingly to him from the future that he abandons his call.

We may summarize the result of this analysis as follows. Past and future are not two absolutely separated regions touching at a highly remarkable zero-point, the name of which is the *present.* Both have a *present* value, they lie contained in the present moment. The past is that which was as it appears to me today, the future is that which comes as it comes to meet me now. (St. Augustine arrived at literally the same conclusion: Conf. XI, 26). Then it is no longer right to define the present as a curious zero-point between two half eternities. The present is a rushing forward. A rushing forward beyond oneself, a being already at and in the things that are to come. And if we ask ourselves *what* it is that rushes forward, what is already with the things to come, then the answer is: that is myself as I became; the present is a throwing forward of what was into what is to come. The present, so we might condense it into a few words, is the going to meet myself as I throw myself as what I have become into the future.* As soon as we have ascertained this, another question arises. How is it that one person throws himself into the future so much discouraged that the going towards this future becomes an arduous task, whereas another places such a very inviting self in the future that life means a pleasant or even eager progress? It will be attempted to find the answer, which for reasons easily understood is of great signification to the psychopathology of the neuroses, by means of two examples.

Of all living beings man is the only one who knows that he *will die. If he wishes to he can see every day that man's life moves towards a usually infirm and difficult old age, followed in most cases by an end full of pain and anguish. A discouraging thought! Even more discouraging if we reflect that death does not at all always*

come when life is rounded off, but may intrude at any moment, in the midst of our
plans, in the midst of life, which must be called unfinished then in every respect.
Death threatens not only as a final ending but hangs over us as a catastrophe that
may strike us down at any moment. If there is one thing that we know with
absolute certainty about the future it is that death will come. It might therefore be
expected that all of us should go to meet this ending with great reluctance, that life
should be to everyone an extremely hesitating, reluctant progress from day to day.
The curious thing however is that very little of this is to be perceived. When we
see people live, when we ask how we ourselves live, then we should be more
inclined to think that hardly anyone takes death into serious consideration. We act
as if there exists no sickly old age, there threatens no painful end, as if death
could not at any moment become a fact to us. A little German poem gives such
perfect expression to this discrepancy:

> / live, I don't know for how long, I die, I don't know when, I
>
> travel, I don't know whither, How strange that 1 am so glad! *

And yet, less strange when we ask the people around us (and ourselves!) for their
opinion about death. As a rule the answer consists in evading the question. They
say: "I don't think about that yet" of "well, that's very simple, one dies when the
time has come." One dies, that is the form of the answer generally given to
oneself to the question about death. One dies, that is the way in which one places
oneself, dying, in the future. The intention is clear. Who says "one dies" has shaken
off all the discouraging elements contained in the consciousness of a certain end.
Where personal death has been transformed into a "one dies," life may safely be
continued "gladly." It is self-evident that this feeling of quiet and gladness is never
quite complete. The quiet of "one dies" is continually undermined by the disquiet of "/
die," the gladness caused by unbroken health is as continually undermined by the
distress at the vulnerability of the body. We must even say that where death and
illness are constantly being turned into the anonymous *"one* falls ill and dies," illness
and death are lurking round the corner of every street, like secret, but by no means
absent enemies.

The camouflage of death and illness has in our times assumed enormous
proportions. Reading J. Huizinga's *The Waning of the hiiddle-Ages* we see how in
those days death and illness were visible to all eyes. The sick were in the streets,
they sat by the side of the road, the lepers used rattles to proclaim their presence.

Death appeared in a guise immediately concerning all, in the death-dance a game was played with death that was clear to all. If anybody died the whole city took part in his funeral by tolling the bell, he was buried under the eyes of all: in the churchyard, situated round the center, the church. Death was there, just as illness. We can very decidedly not say this of our time. The sick are removed from public life, they lie and live in hospitals or in sanatoria. On visiting these medical centers, we perceive very little of illness. There is laughter, singing, hardly anywhere does the visitor meet with suffering. For the seriously sick patients are given separate rooms, they are ill as it were in secret. If death comes, the other patients do not as a rule perceive anything of it directly, there are whispers, like a secret death steals through the room, he may not show himself. To the dying person himself too they wish death—with the best intention of course—to appear under camouflage, the doctor administers morphia; there is very little conscious dying done nowadays. In most cases the churchyard is no more to be found in the center of the town. Out in the country, under a roof of foliage the last resting-place is to be found. One who passes there would sooner expect a splendid country seat than the realm of death. Death has become a camouflaged death, a secret enemy, very carefully rendered invisible.

Very much has been gained in this way of course. It is right, hygienically right, that the sick are no longer wandering up and down the country. It is humane to bestow on them the care due to them, it would be heartless to deprive them of narcotics when the end becomes painful, too painful. But a great loss is threatening as well. Psychologically it is extremely dangerous to banish sickness and death from daily life. Where this happens both become catastrophes taking man by surprise, entirely unprepared. Present-day man is comparable to the young Buddha, who, kept far from any and every form of human suffering by his educators, was unusually vulnerable to everything that was out of keeping with his artificial paradise. It is certainly no matter of chance that in our days so much is thought and written about anxiety. For we are not living with the realities of our existence, we dose our eyes to realities such as illness and death, which through this very denial obtrude themselves to us in the form of an undefined anxiety. Anxiety lies at the bottom of our apparently so joyous life.

If we inquire into the reason why man condenses the whole of his experiences regarding death into the statement "one dies" and then throws it in this anonymous form before him as final future, then the answer is not so difficult. One who reduces his personal death to "one dies" and in this anonymous form throws it before him as final future, need have no further fear that it will come to meet him in the disquieting form of "I die." A heavy burden has in this way been removed from life, life has become easier, more pleasant, in brief more livable. Such was the intention.

It need hardly be said that this solution of the personal problem is not the happiest. A superficial rest is acquired but at the same time a very definite smouldering disquiet. The time of illness and dying may show what fire flares up from this smouldering. We know that this fire not seldom consumes the value of a whole life. That the solution of "one dies" is not a success, is taught by the end: when death comes it becomes dear that it cannot be driven out by an anonymous formula. But life itself brings it even much more sharply home to us that the solution is specious. Where life is not nurtured by the consciousness that it has an undeniable end, that it is "doomed to die," this life becomes superficial and insignificant, it is robbed of something truly human. Man is the only living creature that knows that he is to die. Where this is realized less or no longer, there man is also less man or no longer so.

Summarizing we can say: man chooses the form in which he throws his past before him, he chooses the form in which he places himself in the future. He chooses a similar aspect of the future, that it becomes possible for him to live *on*. A second example may further illustrate this.

In a factory a workman falls from a high ladder and breaks his thighbone. The leg is set in a hospital and after a short time, although it is still difficult for him to walk, he can go home. A certain number of weeks after that the medical officer declares the patient to be all right and the workman resumes work. On that same day, however, he feels that his leg is still very painful. He appears at the consulting hour of the factory doctor, who advises him to work half-time only for the next few weeks. But he cannot manage that either. He is admitted to the hospital for observation, but neither the examination nor the Rontgen photos reveal any deviation. It is therefore decided that the patient is to start work again; he says though that
he is unable to work, stays at home, walks with a limp and complains of his lot to anyone who will listen to him. What has happened here?

We should no doubt learn from a painstaking exploration of the life history of this patient that before his fall he was in a conflict situation. It may be that there is a state of profound dissatisfaction with his work, possibly he is on very strained terms with his employer, possibly he has lost his bearings generally. For our investigation it is unimportant to know where the shoe pinches. It is only important that he is in a conflict situation and that this is interrupted for a short time by his fall from the ladder. We may assume that the workman at the moment of the painful fracture of his leg at the same time heaves a sigh of relief, the meaning of which he will hardly be able to read himself. During the days in the hospital the factory is far away and so are his difEculties, centered in it; no sooner however has his leg recovered than the difficulties come nearer again. Need we wonder that the recovery is slow, that a slight pain is to him a very noticeable pain and that the difficulty in walking at once suggests lameness to him? Surely there is no one who has not gone through a similar experience himself. One who gets up in the morning with a slight headache will in general be much more aware of this headache if he has an unattractive day before him than if it promises a number of pleasant hours. It would not be correct to assume "pretending," gross exaggeration or shamming in the former case. There is no "objective pain." A pain always acquires that magnitude which harmonizes with the whole of life. Which does not mean that the happy do not know pain, it is only that their way of bearing it will differ from that of the unhappy.

What happens to the workman can be expressed in the following words. When after his leg had been set, he was lying in his clean white hospital bed, an important event had been added to his past: the fall and the fracture. The weeks that are coming will undoubtedly be determined by this fact. But how? Here the patient has to "choose." In what form will he place his broken leg in the future? Of course in that form which makes the future appeal to him most strongly. So in the form of an important fact: of severe pain and of great trouble with walking. It might be said that in doing so the patient makes a choice that is most unfortunate for himself: a life of much pain and great lameness (for the pain and the lameness are by no means simulated, they are in a very special sense real, *the patient supers)* is far from attractive. That he makes this choice all the same is caused by the fact that a life of health provides him with quite a different pain and lameness: the pain for in- stance of being continually humiliated and the lameness of a life savouring too much of slavery. And these last mentioned pain and lameness are far more difficult to bear. He therefore chooses rightly. Or rather he does not at all choose rightly, for is not it obviously much better to settle the conflicts in his work or at a pinch look for other work? Sooner said than done however. Who can say how extremely difficult it may be to carry through a change of existence? He chooses the way that is for him the easiest, perhaps the only one. In this case of his fractured leg he is almost compelled to choose that disturbance which will keep him forever far away from his conflict situation. He is—not quite—forced into a—not quite—*free* choice (Sartre).

Let us survey it all once more as follows. The laborer worked in a conflict situation. Suppose conditions in the factory were really awkward for him, we should not forget that he did not very felicitously react to these conditions. Other workmen made a better stand in the same situation. The right way for us to put it is; the relationship of man and situation is a dialogue, the dialogue of workman and factory became a disputation (though there never were any angry words, very probably things would have been much better if there had been). The trauma— the fracture of the leg—acquired its signification from this "disputation": it instantly was a serious trauma, a very serious trauma, the pain was bad, the face of the man who had fallen was markedly distorted with pain, his helplessness clearly visible to all. The trauma had instantly to play a part, as everything in the life of man is thrown forward and has a part to play. The part this trauma had to play was to put an end to the almost unbearable conflict situation. The trauma was to keep the workman far from the factory, far from the argumentative dialogue into which his working there had resulted. In consequence of which the patient does not recover. His leg may recover medically, as long as the conflict situation continues the pain and the lameness continue as well. Therefore we must not look to the leg for the recovery of the patient, but to the foundered dialogue between him and the factory. To the *dialogue:* not only to the hard "words" the factory flings at him, just as much to the no less hard "words" with which he replies.

This line of thought is not new of course. The time when the psychotrauma was regarded as an objectively registrable fact, with the patient helplessly at its mercy, has been left far behind. Who turns over the more recent psychoanalytical publications perceives that an ever increasing importance is attached to the *situation* in which the psychotrauma takes place. The only change phenomenology would introduce into this line of thought would be that the signification of the situation should be even more stressed. The phenomenologist is inclined to say that the situation *makes the psychotrauma possible or calls it into being:* no psychotrauma without a difficult situation. We want to enter a little further into this.

If at the taking down of a biography or during a psychoanalytical treatment it appears that the father of the neurotic plays a very dominating and unsympathetic part, then nothing gives us the right to assume that it was that special father who an objectively controllable bad education hampered Mid still hampers a favorable development of his child. A care-fnfly noted heteroamnesis might very well inform us that the father during the education of his child did not make more than the usual number of mistakes; we may even find that the father made a very good job of it. Neither have we the right to assume that the mistakes that he made notwithstanding— every educator makes mistakes—bore such an offensive character as the patient would have us believe. If, tempted by the manifest sincerity of the patient, we should be inclined all the same to dodbt the data of the heteroamnesis, then there are as a rule toothers or sisters of the patient who—with the same father— <bd oat become neurotic and it is not nearly always a case of the {•beat being the eldest or the youngest child, the only girl or the ooly boy, which might account for this exceptional posi-taoa in the family leading to the also exceptional behavior on the part of the father. If in spite of all this there remains a doubt about the correctness of the heteroamnesis, then we daMaVJ do well to consider that of so many really glaringly badly educated children a relatively small percentage after-watds oocne to the consulting hour of the psychotherapist. With-oat wanting to belittle the importance of a good or a bad

*, we may truly say that we have no right to stamp

as an outcome of education. The only thing that we aoan/ wihesitaJingly conclude from the autoamnesis is that the cvatet between the patient and his father has become seriously disturbed. Of course the father gave occasion to this: he *did* make mistakes (like every father). But the son must have given a. very definite reply: he turned the mistakes into *mis*-f*ter, into gross, irreparable mistakes. In this way there grew an ever extending difference between father and son, and all that from that time happened between them derived its signifi cation from this difference. The disturbed contact determined the nature and the gravity of every happening, turned happenings into psychotraumata. When the patient tells us that the father maltreated him, *he ts speaking the truth,* notwithstanding the fact that a third person would speak of a not quite uncalled for "rap over the knuckles." In this disturbed contact a rap over the knuckles *does* amount to a beating. The disturbed contact turns a rap into maltreatment, a smile into a sneer, a serious remark into inhuman hardness: it *creates* the psychotraumata (though the *stimuli* are never lacking). It has struck me more than once that in cases of marriage difficulties one of the partners spoke of being unable to bear the smell of the other any longer. No sooner were the difficulties a thing of the past, than never a word was said any more about the smell. In a marriage quarrel the smell of the other becomes a stench; for lovers the same smell is the theme for the most heavenly poetry. The contact of two people determines the signification of all that occurs between them, it creates the calibre and the quality of the occurrences.

In other words: the son "chooses" the nature of the rap over his knuckles, he "chooses" everything that takes place between them. From the disturbed contact he is compelled to "choose" freely—and at the same time: how unfreely!—the signification of all occurrences. It is not necessary that the choice of the nature of the occurrences is made at the moment of their occurrence. As a rule it is not even before the period of puberty that this choice takes shape. If this puberty is a failure, that is to say if the dialogue between father and son, which exactly then, during puberty, should be brought to a happy conclusion, degenerates into a hopeless disputation, then with that the nature changes of all the occurrences that ever took place between father and son. I should think that everyone has personally come across some such change. He who falls out with a former friend, usually interprets very much of what happened during their friendship in an entirely new way; a new light, as it is expressed, on what happened before. In the same way the lover interprets everything that took place between him and his fiancee before their falling in love in favor of their love: the lover tries to bring the past into line with the love tie, he discovers the indications of mutual affection in a time when there was not any question yet of this affection and the objectively controllable indications therefore were lacking. Dupre spoke of a *mytbification* of the past in these cases *(Patbologie de l'imag-atatjon et de l'emotivite,* 1925). But surely this name gives a wrong impression of what takes place. The disturbed contact between father and son is no myth at all, no more may the appreciation of the nature of the former occurrences be called a mythification: this change is a change into a new *reality:* that reality that is to say which stands out in the disturbed contact and takes shape. Once more: the patient does not delude him-sdf when speaking of his psychotraumata, he gives a faithful K"^"* of how the past appears to him, how this past *must* appear to him in the contact with his father after it became mhinged. *The* term mythification presumes a past presenting one aspect only: that which would be seen by the cool, impartial outsider at the time when this past happened. Well then, this "impartial" past never and nowhere occurs within the scope of human existence.

Tbe treatment of the patient therefore does not consist in a liberating from the psychotraumata of his youth, it is a liberating from the *meaning* of the psychotraumata *through* the liberating from the disturbed contact with—in this case—his father. During the treatment—we are here obviously speaking of the psychoanalytical treatment—the patient learns to choose differently. In the room of the psychotherapist he repeats his youth, his whole life, and meanwhile it becomes clear to him that this life might as well have been different and therefore may also become different, better. The patient changes his past and in doing so gives a new aspect to the future, from which as we know this past continually comes to meet him.

It is only natural that, at the expense of the psychotherapist, he remains true to his method of choosing that was so detrimental to him before. Unnecessarily too, an objective looker-on will say. No more than it was necessary that formerly he made that choice with regard to his father. Certainly the father gave occasion to this way of choosing: being an educator he had a task of course. The psychotherapist has a task as well. And the words used in the execution of this task will be "misunderstood" for the same reason, he creates the mistakes of the psy-chotherapeutic contact. But there is this great difference now that the psychotherapist by methodical procedure points out to him the peculiarities of his behaviour. He is confronted with the contact disturbance which is the central disturbance of every neurosis. The patient does not at all transfer an affect from the father to the psychotherapist, the neurotic affect with regard to the father and that with regard to the psychotherapist have a common denominator: the contact disturbance generally. That he got to be on bad terms with his father is the evil fruit of his contact disturbance (the detrimental choice of the signification of the events), it is the same contact disturbance which during the treatment drives him into the difficulties of the contact with the psychotherapist.

It will be said that with this reasoning a very great responsibility is devolved on the shoulders of the patient. But do we do anything else when we give a patient psychoanalytical treatment? There is no chance of changing the past any more *as it was,* the patient is grown up now, the father (for instance) has played his part. We cannot alleviate his life as it was lived in the past by changing the circumstances; it is indeed highly possible that, supposing it *WAS* possible for us to change the circumstances of a man's youth even now, it would be of no use to set about changing anything, because it would become quite dear that it was not the fault of the circumstances that tibe patient became neurotic. Every psychotherapist who proposes psychoanalytical treatment to a patient proves by the mere fact of making the proposal that it is the patient himself who most change. He himself must change his attitude towards life, he must free *himself* from the past, *himself* assign another part to tills past. The psychotherapist is nothing but the man through whom this change is accomplished by the patient himself. He does not "cure" the patient, the patient tries with his assistance to arrive at a "being different." But if he can be different— ewty psychoanalytical treatment starts from this supposition— tben indeed he must accept a heavy responsibility. The treatment is always, implicitly, an appeal to this responsibility. It would not only be a terrible blunder, but a fla-untruth as well, if one were to "simply" tell the patient that he is to blame for his neurosis. Things are not as simple as ill tint

TSe remaining question to be answered is, whether, for the - idon of the behavior of the patients, it is necessary to ::_- _T :he hypothesis of *the* *unconscious.* Surveying the pre- - ;es the reader must be struck by the absence of the ~ . • riscious. Yet it is clear that numerous significations ice relationships were discussed that are not clearly seen by man in general and very decidedly not by the patient. It is cor rect to say that surprisingly much of what happens in our life entirety escapes our notice and there is not the slightest objec tion to apply the *adjective* "unconscious" to all that which escapes us. There is much therefore that is unconscious, nothing however that would lead us to assume "an" unconscious *(sub-stanfive!),* which would be supposed to exist as a second reality behind the phantoms of healthy and of neurotic life. There is but one reality: that of life as it is lived. *"The" unconscious,p*

1

that "part" of our personality therefore that, equipped with the most wonderful qualities, is supposed to be able to explain the problem of human life, is the product of a premature cessa tion of the psychological analysis of human existence.

Chapter III

HISTORICAL SURVEY,
SUMMARY DISCUSSION OF

a

PHENOMENOLOGICAL LITERATURE

'N MAY 24th 1798 Ph. Pinel, physician of the Paris asylum for male lunatics *"Bicetre,"* in spite of the gravest warnings from the attendants, entered unarmed the cell of a lunatic and in simple and courteous words promised to put him at liberty provided he behaved in an orderly fashion. The patient was an English captain, who had been chained for 45 years already and who had made himself feared most of all the inmates of the asylum because among other things he had killed one of the attendants. When the patient had at last become convinced that Pinel was in earnest, he promised that he would not make any trouble, whereupon Pinel took off his chains and the patient tottered out of the cell. The whole day he walked about the asylum, pointed delightedly at the sky, which he had not seen for so many years, did not give the slightest trouble and towards evening willingly returned to his cell, where he was greatly pleased to see that a bed had been brought in. He remained for another two years in *Bicetre;* he behaved in an orderly way and history tells us that he assisted the nursing staff at their work to the best of his ability. He was not the only one. Pinel took away the chains from very many patients and very often with the same result, extremely surprising in those days (Cf. *Memoires de l'Academie de Medecine, 1836).*

Pinel has certainly not been the first to make a serious attempt to liberate the psychotical patients from their barbarous existence. But he has undoubtedly been the first whose attempt was crowned with success. If we want to find out what was the cause of this, we should pay careful attention to the year in which his spectacular feat was performed. It was in 1798, in Paris, where since 1789 one of the greatest revolutions known in history was being enacted. The first and foremost device of this revolution was *liberty.* May not it be supposed that the success that attended Pinel's attempt to restore liberty to these patients was achieved without any mishaps, because he was convinced of a very special and entirely new power emanating from the word *liberty?* It was a new outlook on man which made it possible for him to meet the patients in such a way that they did not behave like brute animals but like men, be it then like psychically sick men. For the first time in western culture the question was not the incidental event that a certain physician performed the exceptional, more or less adventurous and undoubtedly risky act of taking their chains off his patients. But the reason why Pinel's action was so important Js that, everybody must clearly have seen this, it argued a new outlook on man, also consequently a new outlook on man psychically disturbed. That his action was a sigp. of a revolution in the ideas about man and psychical illness becomes particularly clear to us, when we see that it was precisely after 1798 that we can first speak of a scientifically justified psychiatry. In 1838 there appears the first book that approaches the problems of insanity in the modern way: Esquirol, the first great "modern" psychiatrist that Europe has known, in that year sets down in a book of two volumes the experiences gained from a couple of decades* serious labor *(Des maladies mentales considered sous rapports medical, hygzenique et medico-legal.* Paris, BailHere, 1838); in the same year, under the influence of the same psychiatrist, the first Bill is passed for the protection of the lot of psychiatrical patients (June 30th 1838).

"Psychiatry," so I was told by the French psychiatrist Henri Ey "was born at the moment when the physician took the chains off the patients." It is difficult to doubt the accuracy of this statement: only when regarding the patients as sick *human beings,* as variants of an existence that always remains *human,* is it possible to meet them with that special interest which has as its fruit such a science as psychiatry.

It should not be thought however that with the action of Pinel's the liberation of the patients was complete. When Wernicke in his *Grundriss dev Psychiatric* (1894) writes that "mental diseases are nothing but brain diseases," then this statement dearly shows that medical and therefore human interest is due to the psychiatrical patient, but at the same time that for the psychiatry of those days the patient did not as yet mean much more than a disturbed body. Again and again the patient had to be freed of chains, though the chains were no longer visible ones, and again and again there resulted a new psychiatry from such a liberation. An exhaustive inquiry would certainly go to prove that every time it was a new outlook on man that preceded the liberation of the patient.

We now live in a time when a serious attempt is being made once more to remove an important chain from the psychiatrical patient. That is the one that is expressed in the nomenclature which up to a short time ago we were accustomed to use for the description of his disturbances. Instead of pronouncing a verdict, such as is contained in the professional terms *projection, conversion, transference* etc.—a verdict which ultimately amounts to a condemnation—we wish to make him to speak for himself. We are not so much interested in how far his faculties differ from ours, we ask for a description of the life that has become reality to the patients. We are trying to find a positive pathography of the patient, which up to a short time ago we nearly exclusively described in negative terms. The result consists in a new psychiatry, whose outlines are already becoming clearly discernible. And it goes without saying that the deepest cause of this new psychiatry is to be found in a change in the outlook on man. A historical review of phenomenology can only then lead to a successful result when we first bring ourselves to a serious account of the changes in the outlook on the world and on man characterizing the culture of the last few decades. We should have to start from a description of the last quarter of the preceding century and of the time then following up to today. During such a survey pertaining to the history of culture very great and essential changes would come to light and it is to be expected that after that it would not be difficult any longer to make the changes in psychiatry readily understood. But for such a very important and certainly illuminating study a large book would be required.

For this reason it seems advisable to relinquish the real history of phenomenology and to consider it sufficient to enumerate the books and articles that have come out, accompanied by a short comment.

To him who wants a rapid and yet not too incomplete survey of the history of phenomenology, who, so we might say, wants to take the phenomenological temperature of psychology and psychiatry in the successive periods, some of L. Binswanger's publications may be recommended. This Swiss psychiatrist who without any exaggeration may be called the father of phenomenological psychiatry has during his fertile life again and again rushed into print and described the state of affairs in lucid words that never missed their mark. In his book: *Probleme der dlgeme'men Psychologic* (Berlin, Springer, 1922, 383 p.) he gives a rounded off review, at a moment exceedingly propitious for this purpose, of the new courses taken by psychology since the beginning of the twentieth century. Their consequences for psychiatry are recorded by him in *Ueber Phaenomenologie (Zeitschrip fur die Gesammte Neurologie und Psychiatrze,* 82, 1923). How great the changes are though undergone by general psychology since that time is shown in Binswanger's great work: *Grundjormen und Erkenntnis menschlichen Daseins* (Zurich, Niehans, 1942, 726 p.) while the psychiatric consequences of these changes were set forth in the following two articles: *Ueber die daseinsanalyttsche Forscbungsrichtung In der Psychiatric (SchiveizeY Arcbiv fur Psychiatrie und Neurologie,* 57, 1946); and: *Daseinsanalytik und Psychiatrie (Ner~ venarzt,* 22, 1951). Whereas these four publications form an excellent introduction into the history of phenomenology and the application of phenomenology in psychiatry, it is in the following discussion that I want to make an attempt to trace the line of development of phenomenology more in detail.

In 1894, there appeared an article which must be considered of paramount importance for the development of the idea of phenomenology. It was from the hand of the wellknown author in the field of cultural history, Wilhelm Dilthey, and bore the title: *Ideen fiber erne beschreibende und zergliedernde Psychologic* (later reprinted in the collected works, vol. V; published by Teubner, Leipsic & Berlin, 1924). In this study Dilthey inquires into the nature of a method in psychology. He is obliged to conclude that in his day this method was almost exdusively derived from the natural sciences. Just as in physics, e.g., they proceeded "dissectingly" in psychology: they tried to isolate the "elements" of psychical life and then attempted from the description of these elements to arrive at the psychology of the .whole of human activity. A striking case in point is Wundt's so-called "element-psychology." (cf. *Grundrhs der Psychologie,* 1896).

What characterizes psychical life, according to Dilthey, is that it is not the isolated element but always the whole of an experience that becomes a reality. One who wants to describe the isolated psychical elements has by this mere fact left the domain of psychology. We should look for a method arising from the object that is to be studied. Since the object of psychology (living man) is always an *entirety,* its method, says Dilthey, should not be *constructive* (i.e., leading up from a part to the whole) but analytical; not synthesizing, but descrip- tive. Accordingly the aim of psychology cannot be an *explanation:* for every explanation tries to reduce into elements; this aim is rather a *description,* an *exposition* or " *hermeneusis":* a faithful narrative of what is seen as a whole direct by man himself. *"Die Natur erklaren wir, das Seelenleben aber verstehen wir"* (we want to and are able to explain nature, we contemplate psychical life however with an understanding look). The aim of psychology is to describe in clear words what is seen— in the beginning mostly only very vaguely— at this first understanding glance. When for instance I see a child cry after losing his toys, this connection is at once clear to me, in the same way as it is at once clear to everybody; if I am a psychologist as well, I shall then try to put into lucid words that which was at once so clear to me. The physiologist however wants to "explain," his wish is to get to know the stimulus that leads the lachrimal gland to secrete etc., explanatory connections all of them, but not of the slightest use to the psychologist to make that appear more clearly what he surveyed in an understanding manner at first glance.

The scholar who first introduced Dilthey's distinction between "explaining from elements" and "understandingly surveying" in psychiatry was Karl Jaspers. In his article *Kausale und "ferstandliche" Zusammenhange zwischen Schicksal und Psycbose bei der Dementia praecox (Schizophrenia), (Zeit-schrip-fur die gesammteNeurologie undPsychiatrie,* 14, 1913), he shows that, in studying schizophrenia for instance, the two methods placed side by side by Dilthey lead to entirely different results, *both valuable,* but of which only the result of the "analyzing" or "descriptive" method may properly be called psychological. Jaspers applied the new method with great success in the entire domain of psychopathology: *Allgememe Psycho-pathologie* (Berlin, Springer, 1st. ed. 1913, 338 p.; 4th. ed. 1946, 748 p.), a book which as a survey of psychopathology may be called almost unsurpassed.

Many others followed Jaspers' example. Very numerous are the publications in which by means of the descriptive, "ver-stehende" methods new fields are opened up. It will be sufficient for me to mention some of the most important: E. Kret-schmer: *Der sensitive Beziehungswahn* (Berlin, Springer, 1918), K. Birnbaum: *Psychopathologische Dokumente* (Berlin, Springer, 1920), H. C. Rumke: *Zur Phanomenologie und Klinik des Glucksgefiihls* (Berlin, Springer, 1924).

The working method put into practice in these studies and leading to such remarkable results, briefly amounted to this that *the completest and most careful description possible was given of what is experienced by healthy or by sick people,* of what "is going on within them." Jaspers calls this the phenom-enological method. Phenomenology, according to his definition, is a description of the psychical phenomena directly experienced inwardly, an exposition of what has been given us introspec-tively or, if it concerns another and the psychical patient in particular, an exposition of what comes to show itself to us intrapsychically *("einfuhlend")* with imperative clarity. This intrapsychical understanding of a fellow man is according to Jaspers always a *suspective understanding:* after all, in his opinion, the inner self of another is never given to us direct: we try to aiter into another's life and ask ourselves what we feel. The suspective understanding therefore of another is always founded on our own inner experience; ultimately, as was already defined by Jaspers, all phenomenology depends on *introspection*[1].

In order to avoid very natural misunderstanding it may be stated emphatically that this phenomenology, the phenomenology therefore of Dilthey-Jaspers, is *not identical* with what the name phenomenology indicates nowadays. The word *phenomenology* has acquired a new meaning. It was Ludwig Bins-wanger who in his important article *Ueber Phaenomenologie* (Zeitschrift fur die gesammte Neurologic und Psychiatric, 82, 1923), made it dear that large fields of psychological and psychopathological labor remain fallow if by phenomenology we understand no more than an accurate description of "intra-psychical experiences." In this connection Binswanger pointed to the work of Edmund Husserl: *Logische Untermckungen* (Halle, Niemeyer, 1900-1901), in which the latter continued the work of his teacher F. Brentano: *Psychologic vom empiri-schen Standpunkt* (Leipsig, Duncker & Humblot, 1874), and gave a new meaning to the word. I think it would be of some importance to go into this more fully.

In his *Psychologie* Brentano distinguishes physical and psychical phenomena. He answers the question as to what is characteristic for the psychical phenomena by pointing out that, in contradistinction to the physical phenomena, they are characterized by *being directed toward an object,* by what he called, following the scholastics, *intentionality.* "Every psychical phenomenon encompasses something as its object, although not always in the same way. In the representation something is represented, in a judgment something is accepted or rejected, in love something is loved, in hatred hated, in desire desired, and so on. This intentional 'inexistence' is characteristic of all psychical phenomena, none excepted. Not a single physical phenomenon has anything like it. So that we can define the psychical phenomena by saying: they are those phenomena which intentionally encompass an object within themselves" *(Psychology,* vol. I, p. 125). By the word "inexistence" Brentano wants to indicate that the intentionality does *not* encompass the object itself. In doing so, he sticks to the separation of subject and world: he cannot admit that the intentionality reaches the object itself.

It is Husserl who enters a protest against this reservation. In his *Logiscke Untersuchungen* Husserl says that "it should be possible for anyone to understand that the intentional object of for instance the image is *the same* as the real one, to be found in the outside world and that it is wrong to make any distinction between them" (vol. II, p. 425). In his *Ideen zu einer reinen Phanomenologie* (vol. I, 1913, p. 186) Husserl puts it, if possible, even more clearly. If we should want to separate the object of the outside world from the "immanent," "subjective" "inexistent" object, then, Husserl formulates, "we get into the difficulty that In that case there are *two* realities facing each other, whereas there is only one present and possible. The thing, the 'natural object' is observed by me: the tree yonder in the garden, that and nothing else is the real object of the observing intention." This remark came to be of great importance. It made clear that the rigid distinction between subject and object, between I and the world is an artificial one, that this distinction suggests a very decided, and by no means necessary, philosophical attitude. Of how much importance all this is for psychology and for psychopathology becomes dear to us when we consider that Brentano's intentionality is not only directed towards the other thing, but also towards the other man, the fellow-man, so that Husserl's remark that we observe the thing directly should be equally applicable to the other man: *we observe the other person directly.* The insurmountable distinction *man and fellow man* is as artificial as that between man and object. We "don't find out about the other" via the interpretation of his visible behaviour, *but see him directly.* This is indeed Husserl's opinion. The other is not hidden behind his bodily appearance, no: he shows his inner self in his body, he is visible in his bodily behavior. I shall return to this presently. For it is necessary to dwell for a moment on the considerations that Husserl expresses when he says that observation gives me the object itself. Which object? he asks. It is obvious that things may appear to me in completely different ways. There are different ways of observing. There exists, as he formulates 4, a sensory and a categorial observation *(smnliche und kate-fgoriale Anschauung,* cf. *Logische Untersuchungen,* V. I, P. 2, Ch. 6, pp. 128ff.). "Of every observation it can be said that it 'takes' its object itself or directly. But this direct taking of the object has a different meaning, according as the objectivity taken directly is a sensuous or a categorial one, in other words: according as this object is a real or an ideal one" (L.U., p. 145). Every object can appear either actually or ideally, in the first case the object is "taken" directly or is itself present ("direkt erfasst oder selbst gegenwartig," p. 145), in the second case it is present as "an object of a higher order" ("Gegenstand hoherer Ordnung," L.U. p. 147), which Husserl calls *essence* in his *Ideen:* "Wesen oder Eidos": "the observation can be changed into a seeing of essences. What is observed is then the correlative pure essence or eidos" *(Ideen,* p. 10). Husserl illustrates this by means of an example: "in this way every tone that is heard for example contains the essence of this tone and ultimately the general essence "tone as such," or better still "the acoustic as such" as that which can be recognized as the general tone character from the individual that strikes my ear. In the same way everything has its essence and ultimately the general essence "materiality," with "time specification/' "duration," "space," etc. *(Ideen,* p. 9).

This distinction, i.e., of a sensory and a categorial observation, is endorsed by Binswanger in his article *Ueber Phaenome-nologie.* Binswanger begins with the observation that a natural-scientific bent, which so highly characterizes us all nowadays, divides the reality in which we live into two domains, namely the domain of the material facts and the domain of the psychical ones (cf. Descartes' distinction between *corpus sive res extensa* and *mens she res cogitans).* In accordance with this we should also distinguish two forms of observation: the "external observation" or extrospection and the "internal observa- tion" or introspection (cf. John Locke's distinction of *sensation* and *reflection).* Another, third way is not known to natural science, Binswanger rightly says. And yet there is such a third way, as original, as primary as the other two: the categorial observation, as Husserl distinguishes it from the sensory (internally or externally sensory) observation. It must not be concluded from this that Husserl held the opinion that the categorial observation did not take place by means of our ordinary senses. The appellation "sensory" or "categorial" gives rise to this misunderstanding. No, what Husserl means by his categorial observation is an observation *by means of our senses* although simultaneously with that very special attitude or expectation which is not burdened with the inheritance of Descartes' and Locke's distinctions. The categorial observation, says Binswanger, is "a seeing with the eye and nevertheless a direct perception, a 'regarding' or 'contemplating' whose convincing power is no smaller than that of the 'ordinary' sensory observation but perhaps rather the contrary." It is the observation of the artist, who sees more and "better" than the lens of the camera. A direct observation, of what is really should also characterize the psychologist in his work. For psychology has its being in the margin between sensory and categorial observation. What the artist sees *more* than the lens, *that* is the domain of psychology. The lens sees what has been reduced to a "natural," to an "objective" state, the lens sees what we see "on closer view" (this was our formulation in the preceding chapters) : what we see when what is psychological has been wiped out in what we observed.

This categorial observing consists, says Binswanger, in an "entering into what is observed" ("sich einleben, hineinverset-zen, statt einzelne Merkmale oder Eigenschaften abheben und aufzahlen"). Nevertheless this "entering into what is observed" is not identical with the "understandingly surveying" or the *"Verstehen"* suggested by Jaspers. Where it was Jaspers' opin loo *that* the contact with things and with our fellow men could art roe above an ultimate introspective experiencing of all that winch I experience when I try to put myself in the place of the other thing or the other person, Husserl and Binswanger dissolve his reservation by the documented statement that the fawner between man and his environment is in a certain way, •Oft-existent, that man in a certain way is his environment and out IB consequence of this he can freely approach, not ob-*bf* anything, that which presents itself to his eye—so it is under categorial observation. Here Binswanger

> • the first place as a matter of course of the psychiatrical I don't know the other "suspectively," but observe him

•. To remark that this is impossible is to think exclusively observation, the observation of the lens, the observa-«f the "on doser inspection," which always results in an and which in consequence makes the fellow man he who is "hidden within his body" and "who is not a» be faown." The categorial observation however gives me far other directly. It is out of the question that the lover sus-his beloved behind the screen "body," no: he sees her the face and in the eye there before him—though he that of *this* seeing the lens can record exceedingly

Biaswanger wishes the psychiatrist to "see" in this wiy and he wants him to make a true report of this As a result the psychiatrist is taken step by step into the of the patients ("auf Schritt und Tritt in die Welt "). Binswanger gives some striking cases in point, the best of which is not to be found in this article—which aims other at drawing up a working-plan—but in his study *Ueber Ueemfmcbt,* to which I will presently return.

For I judge it important to go further for a moment into the consequences of Hussed's remarkable tenet that the other can be seen *dtrectly.* We find this tenet in his *Logische Unter- suchungen* (II, 1, p. 34), when the expression is subjected by him to an investigation. He there says: "the understanding of the expression is in no way like an understanding knowledge of the expression, in no way like a judging: it amounts to this, that the hearer *intuitively* considers or rather *observes* the speaker as the person who says so and so. The hearer observes that the speaker gives expression to certain experiences and in the same measure does he himself also observe these experiences."

I am now going to proceed to enumerate the publications that are characterized by phenomenology as it was re-defined by Husserl and Binswanger.

The two studies showing to how great advantage the new orientation can be applied to the psychological interpretations of the *life history* of the well and the sick were: L. Binswanger: *Lebensjunktion und innere Lebensgeschichte (Monatschrift fur Psychiatrie und Neurologic,* 68, 1928); E. Straus: *Gescheb-nis und Erlebnis* (Berlin, Springer, 1930, 129 pp.). It is unfortunately not possible otherwise than by simply mentioning them, to refer to the excellent works that had for their subject matter a phenomenological investigation into the normal and the disturbed human *space* and *time.* The main ones were the following: V. E. Von Gebsattel; *Zeitbezogenes Zwangsdenken in der Melancholic (Nervenarzt,* 1, 1928); E. Straus: *Das Zeit-e-rlebnis in der endogenen Depression und in der psychopat-ischen Verstimmung. (Monatscbrift fur Psychiatric und Neurologie, 68,* 1928). Independent of each other these two psychiatrists give a remarkably similar report of their phenomenological investigation into the "depressive time." Ten years later there appears from both authors another article, this time about the physiognomy of the world of the obsession neurotics, again showing a remarkable similarity in results, *viz.:* V. E. Von Gebsattel: *Die Welt der Zwangskranken (Monatscbrift fur Psychiatric und Neurologic, 99,* 1938); E. Straus: *Ein Bettrag zu¥ Pathologic der Zwangserscheinungen (Monat-schrijt fur Psychiatric und Neurologic,* 98, 1938), while the latter somewhat earlier described the possibilities of a phenom-enologie of human space already in an absorbing article: E. Straus: *Die Formen des Raumlichen (Nervenarzt,* 3, 1930), the main line of thought of which he worked out at greater length in the book that well deserves to be called a standard work now; E. Straus: *Vom Sinn der Smne* (Berlin, Springer, 1935, 314 p.). As the title of the book suggests the author is trying to find a new psychology of the senses, which, as indeed is to be expected now, proves to consist in a new psychology of the 'perceptible) world.

The author who first applied the Husserl-Binswanger phenomenology to the group of the schizophrenic disturbances was F. Fischer. Of his many publications we will mention only the fallowing two, of which the first is specially concerned with lie psychopathology of schizophrenic time and the second has is its subject schizophrenic space: F. Fischer: *Zeitstruktur und* (Zeitschrift fur die gesammte Neurologie und 121, 1929); F. Fischer: *Ueber die Wandlungen da Spates tm*

Aufbau der sckizophrenen Erlebniswelt (Ner- 1934).

We see in an isolated position, also owing to the fact that *sztbat* worked in Paris for many years, the far too little book by Minkowski, which makes a serious and in many r successful attempt to understand psychopathology the disturbances in time-experience: E. Minkowski: *Le* (Paris, Artrey, 1933, 401 pp.). In this same year 1933 however there appears a book which clearly shows in fcpv *far* the works just mentioned did not yet take the last of Husserl's starting point. Again it was Binswanger, who in his pathography of a maniacal patient gives a exposition of the signification of the world in which the lives and realizes himself as a manic disturbed man: *Ueber Ideenftucht* (Zurich, Fiissli, 1933, 214 p.; this work first appeared in the form of two articles in the *Schwetzer Archh -fur Psychiatric und Neurologie,* 28-29, 1931-1932).

It is remarkable that this work is also preceded by a philosophical work written by a pupil of Husserl's clearing the way for a new and also original description of human existence. It was: M. Heidegger: *Sein und Zeit* (Halle, Nlemeyer, 1927, 438 pp.). Binswanger's publication is the direct consequence of this pioneering work.

So we see three periods in the history of phenomenological psychiatry. The first period was ushered in by Jaspers (1913), the two following by Binswanger (1923, 1933), each period being preceded by a new, philosophical reflection about the nature of human existence (by Dilthey, Husserl and Heidegger respectively). If there is a marked difference between the first and the second period regarding the meaning of the name phenomenology, the two latter periods merge so harmoniously into one another, that no alteration is necessary in the original meaning of the word as it had been defined by Husserl.

A little more than ten years later there appears also from Binswanger's hand the first comprehensive phenomenological pathography of a patient suffering from a special form of schizophrenia: *Der Fall Ellen West (Schweizer Archh fur Psychiatric und Neurologie,* 53-55, 1945), quickly followed by three other studies, also concerning schizophrenia (all three by Binswanger): *Wahnsinn als lebensgeschichtliches Phanomen und als Geisteskrankheit (Monatschrift fur Psychiatric und Neurologie,* 110, 1945,) *Der Fall Jurg Ziind (Schweizer Archh fur Psychiatric und Neurologie,* 56-59, 1947), *Der Fall Lola Voss (Schwefaer Archiv jar Psychiatric und Neurologic,* 63, 1949).

Binswanger's pupil Roland Kuhn wrote the first phenomenological pathography of a sexually disturbed person: *Analyse eines Mordversuches eines depressiven Fetischisten und Sod- omisten cm einer Dime (Monatschrift fur Psychiatrie und Neurologic,* 116, 1946), and another Swiss psychiatrist tried to devise an entire pathosexuology on a new basis: M. Boss: *Sinn und Gehalt der sexuellen Perversionen* (Bern, Huber, 1947, 130pp.).

The Dutch psychiatrist Van Der Horst and his pupils attempted to describe, successfully In many respects, the greater part of psychiatry from a phenomenological standpoint: L. Van Der Horst, c.s.: *Anthropological Psychiatry* (2 vols., Amsterdam, Holkema & Warendorf, 1946, 790 pp.).

One more word about the changes that took place in France. In that country there also appeared an important philosophical work that struck a highly responsive chord: J. -P. Sartre. *L'etre et If neant* (Paris, Gallimard, 1943, 724 pp.). In this work the mfloence of Husserl and Heidegger is clearly to be felt; the book famishes excellent examples of phenomenological insight. Especially the chapters on the human look and on the body may be courted among the best ever written in the field of phenomenology. Curiously enough French psychiatry has hardly been influenced up till now by this work. All the more curious because French psychology was remarkably strongly influenced by it. Though it is beyond the scope of this book I cannot refrain from mentioning here the names of some leading French psychologists vfaose work has been strongly coloured by Sartre's existential-istic philosophy: Merleau-Ponty, Jeanson, SImone De Beauvoir, Moodier and Gusdorf. The last mentioned has given us in his *L decomrerte de sot* (Paris, Presses universitaires de France, 19^8, 513 pp.) a book which possesses priceless values as the chief feature of a new psychology.

Special mention should also be made of the work of Gaston Bachelard. Though not visibly influenced by the new currents in the German and the French philosophy he designed a psychology of the elements fire, water, air and earth, as can solely be written by a phenomenologist. In my opinion his publications are of immediate signification for psychopathology. For is it not very often that a patient tells us that he is in an entirely new position with regard to the elements of his existence? It is of great importance that Bachelard made a serious attempt to expound their meaning in the life of the man in good health. I will therefore mention the following of his publications: *La psychanalyse du feu* (Paris, Gallimard,

1938, 220 pp.); *L'&au el les reves* (Paris, Corti, 1942, 265 pp.)'> *L'air et les songes* (Paris, Corti, 1943, 306 pp.); *La terre et les reveries de la volonte* (Paris, Corti, 1948, 407 pp.); and *La terre et les reveries du repos* (Paris, Corti, 1948, 337 pp.). Now that I do find myself for a moment in the field of phenomenological *psychology,* I will not omit mentioning two more authors who certainly showed that the phenomenological method can lead in their province to remarkable results: O. F. Bollnow, who published in 1943 his book on the moods *(Das Wesen der Stimmungen,* Frankfurt a.M., Klostermann, 255 pp.), and the Dutch psychologist F. J. J. Buytendijk, who by a series of excellent articles and books rendered a great service to Dutch phenomenological psychology.

Finally I must mention the French psychotherapist R. Desoille, the framer of a phenomenologically orientated psychotherapy. I have availed myself of his renovating thought in the paragraph on the life history in this book. His most important publications are the following: *La veve eveille en psychotherapte* (Paris, Presses universitaires de France, 1945, 388 pp.); *Psychanalyse et reve eveille dmge* (Bar-le-Duc, Comte-Jacquet, 1947, 93 pp.).

EPILOGUE

P /CHIATRY IS A MEDICAL science. It has its origin in the fact that there are :k, helpless people. It arises from the need to help the sick man to the best of one's ability. The psychiatrist wishes to help. The special quality of his help however lies in the fact that it is not a disturbed organ or a disturbed function that is concerned, but a disturbed personality. The psyehiatri-cally sick man is always ill in his entirety, his illness is a form of being. The psychiatrist wants to help a *man*. But what does this amount to? What does it mean that the psychiatrist has the intention *to help* a man, a human existence, a human existence that has in a special way come to a deadlock? It seems difficult to answer this question which is so easily asked. For as simple as it is to say what the medical help means that is *not* intended for the entire man, so difficult it is to indicate even to a slightly elucidating extent what psychiatrical help in the end amounts to. The dermatologist notes a deviation of the organ *skin,* he makes the diagnosis, he knows the appropriate therapy, he professionally applies it and the patient allows all this to be done pretty much "as if he himself were not there." He shows his skin as a part of his body that shows undesirable changes, as a disturbed object, a *thing,* and he lets the physician treat this disturbed thing in much the same way as he has the painter inspect and paint his weather-stained house. The surgeon notices a deviation with the appendix, he makes the diagnosis "acute infection," knows the appropriate action and operates: in this case too the patient is only indirectly concerned- Not he himself is ill, but his appendix, a part of his body, a *thing,* for which he certainly calls in professional, but definitely not personal, help. The surgeon who attends him need not be congenial to him, need not mean anything to him as a man, he requires in the first place a skillful surgeon. It need not be said that such an only-skillful dermatologist a«,,. such an exclusively-technical surgeon are not the best examples of a physician in the true sense of the word. As a rule the dermatologist and the surgeon are incomparably "more" than that. The physician, if he is really good at his business, is a human being, who meets his patient in the first place "humanly" and attends to him professionally and skillfully into the bargain. We might formulate it also thus; the physician is always something like a psychiatrist as well; also in those cases where his medical help means technical treatment of the disturbed organ. Before he examines the organ with a clinical eye and touches it with a physician's hand, before he seizes the medicament or the knife, he has listened to the patient, he has come to meet him, he has *helped* him already. What is this helping? What is the secret of this helping which has become the absolute main purpose in psychiatry?

About 1800 the Danish philosopher Soren Kierkegaard asked himself the same question and he found an answer that must be called exemplary.

The secret of all helping, thus Kierkegaard expresses it, lies in the fact that he who wishes to lead a person to a special aim, i.e., wants to help a person—must realize with great precision, to look for the person needing help there where he really is, and to begin there where he is found. This means: to help is before everything to put oneself in the other's place, to make one's home in his existence, to learn to know the world in which he lives. Undoubtedly to help is not: to dictate a way to the person needing help without knowing or even wanting to know whether the way dictated can join up with his existence. To help is: to enter the existence that is the other's.

In phenomenological psychiatry these words of Kierkegaard's have acquired a new sense again. The phenomenologist tries to give a description of the world that has become reality for the patient. He wants to know the physiognomy of the things as it strikes his patient. Putting it more simply: he wants to completely understand his existence before he ventures to judge of this existence. And the one aim is: to help the patient. Or rather, by completely realizing what the patient's existence is, what his world looks like, he has already, so he trusts, offered to the patient that form of help which is the foundation for all further help.

It will be said that this is anything but new. So it is, to be sure. Helping in a medical way has always been founded on the serious endeavour to seek the fellow man and to try and find where he is. Psychoanalysis shows us in an exemplary fashion that no effort is ever spared to arrive at a thorough penetration and understanding of the patient's existence. The one new thing in phenomenological psychiatry lies in the fact that the way of helping which as we saw was always practised in the medical situation is investigated in a new way. Phenomenological psychiatry does not profess a new method of curing, k only says in new words what at all times and in all countries was the foundation of this human occupation *par excellence:* that the healthy man assists the sick in word and deed.